Feed Your Brain
Lose Your Belly

Other books by Larry McCleary, MD

The Brain Trust Program
(2007, Perigee Press)

Bald Is Beautiful:
The Shining Stars Foundation Guide
for Living with Childhood Cancer
(2009)
(Available at www.ShiningStarsFoundation.com)

Feed Your Brain
Lose Your Belly

Larry McCleary, MD

ISBN 978-0-615-33950-4

A Publisher's Note: Neither the publisher nor the author is engaged in rendering professional advice or services to the individual reader. The ideas, procedures and suggestions contained in this book are not intended as a substitute for consulting with your physician. All matters regarding your health require medical supervision. Neither the author nor the publisher shall be liable or responsible for any loss or damage allegedly arising from any information or suggestion in this book. The names and identifying characteristics of patients and persons interviewed have been changed to protect their privacy.

Interior design by Sue Knopf

To Heather, Luke, Mike and Stella

Contents

Part 1: The Brain–Belly Connection

Part 2: Brain and Belly Friendly Diets

Part 3: Training Your Brain to Lose Your Belly

Part 4: How We Know the Brain–Belly Connection Really Works!

Acknowledgments

I would like to acknowledge the invaluable contributions made in the preparation of this manuscript by Christine McCleary.

Introduction

Exploring how what we eat affects our health has always been an interest of mine—especially when it involves the brain. As a pediatric neurosurgeon, I witnessed firsthand how good nutrition sped up the recovery of some very sick young brains suffering from head trauma, bleeding and even brain tumors.

The same applies to older brains. It is well known that eating a healthy diet slows brain aging. However, what is not generally appreciated is that memory loss, difficulty thinking and even Alzheimer's disease are associated with "brain starvation." Scientifically speaking this refers to an inability of the brain to properly take up and use glucose (its major fuel source). Under such circumstances, it's as if the brain is not getting enough nutrition. As a result since it can't generate the energy it needs to produce all the electrical signals it requires to function properly, it suffers the equivalent of a power outage. These electrical "brownouts" contribute to the development of mental fatigue, difficulty concentrating, "senior moments" and, as mentioned above, are even being scientifically linked with more ominous conditions.

Alzheimer's disease and other so-called dementing disorders have increased exponentially during the past several decades. Over the same time period we have seen an explosion in the number of cases of obesity and diabetes—even in children! In this context the question that was puzzling to me was, "How can our brains be starving while we're overfeeding our bodies?" It just didn't make sense.

It seemed to me that many of the calories we were consuming somehow bypassed our brains and ended up being stored in fat cells. I began wondering whether there might be a relationship between the rise in brain problems and our expanding waistlines. And, if so, what we could do about it.

However, several years passed before I was able to better understand the connection between the two. Coincidently, at that time a young patient of mine developed diabetes shortly after her sixth birthday. As a result she had to self-administer insulin (the hormone that controls blood sugar levels) by giving herself injections four times a day. One morning as I entered the hospital, I noticed her name on the patient board in the Emergency Room. She had injected too much insulin at dinner the night before and had blacked out and suffered several convulsions. These were due to the fact that her blood sugar level had plummeted (due to the inadvertent insulin overdose) and *literally starved her brain!* Not receiving enough glucose has the same effect on the brain as not getting enough oxygen—it stops working properly and this can happen suddenly.

By too rapidly clearing glucose from her bloodstream her insulin overdose produced hypoglycemia (low blood sugar). It is well known to endocrinologists (hormone doctors) that insulin controls blood sugar by transporting glucose out of the blood into various other cells throughout the body (and *away* from brain cells). This shortage literally starved her brain and resulted in her seizures and loss of consciousness. That is when it dawned on me that elevated insulin levels might play a key role in both the fattening of America and the brain starvation being seen in aging brains!

As I investigated this potential connection it became clear that there *were* links between memory loss and problems controlling blood glucose levels. Medical journal articles were being published that documented associations of obesity and diabetes with memory problems and even Alzheimer's disease. It appeared as if becoming overweight or developing diabetes were *risk factors* for the development of some common brain disorders! But how could this connection be explained?

That morning encounter in the ER provided insight into what I had been struggling with for a while! Could insulin—a hormone that is considered to be merely a blood glucose regulator—be the key to understanding a host of brain *and* body diseases? That's when I realized that elevated insulin levels might explain the diversion of food calories from our brains to our bellies, much like insulin shunted glucose away from my young patient's brain to other cells in her body!

There was one additional piece of the puzzle that needed to be understood. How could elevated insulin levels contribute to expanding waistlines? As we shall see, there is an obvious explanation—the development of what I refer to as "sticky fat cells!" They play a pivotal role in the fattening process by storing calories in ways that prevent them from being easily accessed and, in so doing, inappropriately triggering our appetite centers. High insulin levels trick fat cells into becoming sticky.

These observations eventually helped me understand how brains and bellies are related; what role sticky fat cells play; why calories in the food we eat bypass our brains and end up making us get fat in the process; and what role our daily food choices play.

Being a brain surgeon gave me a unique perspective of this brain–belly interaction and helped me connect the dots, as it were, in making sense of such seemingly unrelated findings. This knowledge culminated in the writing of *Feed Your Brain Lose Your Belly*.

It also made me realize that forcing ourselves to eat less is *not* the solution to either problem—*avoiding the development of sticky fat cells is*. Based on these insights, I now believe that *what* we eat is the primary reason we are in the midst of an epidemic of both obesity and Alzheimer's disease. The simple solution to these worldwide problems is to learn how to properly feed our brains while simultaneously starving our bellies—just the opposite of what many of us are doing.

To determine how well the dietary approach that I developed based on these observations—the Feed Your Brain Lose Your Belly diet program—worked, it was formally tested on a group of human volunteers in a clinical trial setting. The results of that testing are fully discussed in Chapter 11.

To better understand this dilemma, learn why it occurs and how to easily reverse the process, I encourage you to keep reading to discover what you must do to preserve the health of your brain and body.

Larry McCleary, M. D.
Incline Village, NV
2010

Part 1
The Brain–Belly Connection

1

"Built-in Pantries"

In March, 1963, newspapers around the world described the almost incredible story of the seven weeks deprivation of food and the survival of Ralph Flores, a forty-two-year-old pilot of San Bruno, California, and twenty-one-year-old Helen Klaben, a co-ed of Brooklyn, New York, following a plane crash on a mountainside in Northern British Columbia. The couple was rescued March 25, 1963, after forty-nine days in the wilderness in the dead of winter, over thirty days of this time without any food at all. ...

Miss Klaben, who was "pleasing plump" at the time of the plane crash, was happily surprised, at the ordeal's end, to learn that her weight loss totaled thirty pounds.

Flores, who was more physically active during their enforced fast, had lost forty pounds. Physicians who examined them after the rescue found them to be in "remarkably good" condition.

FROM "LIVING WITHOUT EATING" (ARTICLE #1)

BY DR. HERBERT M. SHELTON

The interesting question that arises from this observation is not how long man can survive a fast, but what enables him to do so. All the hallmarks of life such as movement, thought, heartbeat and digestion do not magically halt during a fast—regardless of whether it is voluntary or enforced.

The body normally must prepare itself for such an unintended happenstance. If not, all the evolutionary prowess that resulted in man's preeminent stature in the animal kingdom would have been for naught. Neither man nor animal can survive prolonged abstinence without a readily accessible store of reserve food (our fatty tissue) to tide him over. Many observations have confirmed the fact that when an organism goes without eating, the bodily tissues are sacrificed as a source of energy in reverse order of their importance. Hence, fat is the first to go. Herein lies the importance of fat stores—our "built-in pantries."

In *The Guinness Book of World Records*—Not!

The most extraordinary records of continued abstinence from food are found among the lower animal species. Compared to them, man is a neophyte. The time vertebrates (animals with backbones) can survive without eating ranges from a few days in small birds and mammals to a few years in reptiles. The exact duration depends on the amount of food reserve present and the rate at which it is consumed.

In cold-blooded animals the demands made on the nutritional reserves are usually minimal, so they may fast for long intervals. In warm-blooded animals like humans, reserves are frequently lower and demands are higher. Thus, survival without food is usually shorter. Survival time in cold-blooded animals is longer because they are not required to "burn fuel" in order to maintain their body temperature.

Invertebrates (animals without backbones) can withstand even more prolonged periods of starvation. It has been documented that larvae of the *Trogderma tarsale* have survived *for five years*, during which time they lost 99.8% of their body substance!

With a circulation of blood active enough to maintain their body temperature up to one hundred degrees above that of the surrounding environment, bears and badgers can dispense bodily food stores over periods of three to five months in such a manner that they emerge in full possession of their "physical and mental energies."

Compared to the seemingly Herculean feats of fasting described above, man is not even in the same league. As was described for the survivors of the 1963 plane crash, thirty days without food made headlines around the world.

This is primarily because man is warm-blooded (meaning he has to continuously burn calories to maintain a higher body temperature) and has a large, energy-hungry brain.

An Inability to Store Calories Is Associated with a Short Lifespan

Many insects that have an extraordinarily brief life share the phenomenon of fasting during the mating season. Caterpillars do little other than eat. However, after they become butterflies they usually never eat again. Some insects actually have no provision for hunger and are devoid of digestive organs when fully developed. Ephemera species (mayflies) come into the world in the evening; mate; the female lays her eggs and by morning both sexes are dead. Destined for little more than reproduction, *they have no mouths and do not eat!*

Hence, in the insect kingdom a mouth and an appetite appear to be necessary for survival and longer lives. The same is true for humans.

Humans cannot fast long compared to some other animals because they are warm-blooded and must continuously burn calories to maintain a high body temperature and feed their large, energy-hungry brains.

Warm-Blooded and Smart!

It is clear that an inability to store food energy in a portable fashion through "built-in pantries" is associated with poor long-term survival. Yet, being born human saddles us with two major obstacles that conspire to make fat storage difficult—being warm-blooded and having a big brain. A large energy demand is the price we pay for these characteristics.

While that is true, they both provide unique benefits. It is this balancing act that we must contend with. What is good in one situation can be detrimental in another. The warm-blooded state exists at the expense of a higher and more energetically costly metabolic rate, which means we need to burn more calories our entire life. When food is scarce, this can be a real problem. The trade-off is that by maintaining a higher stable temperature, all of the chemical reactions in the body run in a more predictable and well-coordinated fashion.

Even during sleep a large brain consumes calories ten times faster than the rest of the body. This also puts us at risk during times of famine. But big brains have obvious advantages that make such a compromise worthwhile in the long run.

The Brain and the Mouth

In most species roaming the planet, there is an almost fixed and close relationship between the location of the mouth and the brain. This is no coincidence! The brain is very concerned about what the mouth is doing and has a vested interest in what goes into it. By being the repository of the appetite centers, the brain controls how hungry we are and how much we eat. The mouth is the portal of entry for all of this food.

The brain must also monitor dietary contents for any toxic "foods" that might cause ill effects. This is so important for the brain that, unlike any other organ, it is surrounded by a well-developed protective membrane called the blood-brain-barrier

(BBB) whose job it is to prevent access to the brain cavity of any chemicals that might harm the 100 billion or so nerve cells that make up the most powerful thinking machine in nature.

There are other vital reasons the brain–mouth relationship is so important. Unlike other bodily organs, such as muscles and the heart, which can generate the power they depend upon from a diversity of nutrient fuels, the brain doesn't have that luxury. It must rely on the burning of glucose (the "sugar" in blood) as its only source of energy.

Not only that, but the brain can't store nutrients the way the body can. When blood sugar levels fall, it can go for only a few seconds before it suffers from an "energy brownout" and we lose consciousness. Herein lies the significance of the brain–mouth connection.

The Importance of the "Built-in Pantries"

Make no mistake, the ability to store energy when we don't know where the next meal is coming from—or if it will ever arrive —is vital for survival. Not only that, but imagine what life would be like if we weren't able to store the energy from food and had to eat continuously. Sleep and many other functions would be impossible. So, whether it involves getting from breakfast to lunch or surviving a famine, the ability to store food energy and other nutrients internally and to be able to carry them around with us is a real lifesaver!

Our ability to store energy when we don't know where our next meal is coming from is vital for survival.

The Brain–Belly Connection

When we get hungry, it's really not an empty stomach but rather our brain telling us to eat more. The brain performs its vital duties in conjunction with our "belly," or, more appropriately, the collection of adipose tissue (fat cells) around our middle. This continual dialogue is our lifeline during periodic food shortages. It is also what gets us from meal to meal. So, whether we don't eat for a few hours or a few weeks, our belly is an important player.

Unlike the Ephemera species that has no mouths or intestines, we have the luxury of accessing nutrients from both *internal* and *external* sources. Our fat tissue represents the main repository of our internal energy stores. What we eat constitutes the external energy supply. When one is absent, we rely on the other. The Brain–Belly Connection orchestrates this interaction. It does so by controlling the hunger response and overseeing what the mouth eats.

Hormones

At one time or another we have all heard someone who has gained a few pounds lamenting the fact that it must be due to a hormonal problem. Hormones are the master conductors of many bodily functions including puberty, menopause, reproduction and how we respond to stress as well as a host of metabolic pathways. Due to its well-known ability to speed up or slow down the rate at which we burn calories, thyroid hormone is the hormone that usually comes to mind when weight concerns arise. Unfortunately, it is rarely a significant factor in the "battle of the bulge."

Hormones are chemical compounds that are produced by certain cells in the body and are released into the bloodstream. They float around until they come into contact with their "target" cells—cells that have receptors on their surface that enable them to "hook up" with a specific hormone. This hand-and-glove

Hormones are the master conductors of many bodily functions including puberty, menopause, reproduction and how we respond to stress as well as a host of metabolic pathways.

interaction is what triggers the desired changes to take place within the target cell. For example, it is how thyroid hormone is able to speed up heart rate when it binds to the nerves that control heartbeat.

If thyroid hormone is not usually the cause when we gain five or ten pounds, then what is the culprit? Another hormone? To answer this question, we must first understand how the body stores fat and what allows it to build up in unwanted ways.

As we have learned, fat is a storage form of energy that is portable—meaning that if we find ourselves in the middle of a food shortage, we can utilize the bodily fat we carry around with us. For the system to work properly, we must be able to store excess calories as fat *but also to access them when required*. After all, if we can't use them when we need to, what good are they? The ability to easily avail ourselves of the fat stored in our built-in pantries is a concept that has not received proper attention in the ongoing weight gain, weight loss discussion among experts.

This is where hormones come into play. They determine whether we are in a fat-storing or a fat-burning mode. Hormonal messengers act like translators that relay signals between various body organs so that they are all on the same page when called upon to respond. Two organs with which hormones interact to coordinate this delicate balance are the brain and fat tissue.

Fat Storage

The ability to store the energy from food as fat is a carefully controlled process that has allowed us to survive for millions of years under inhospitable conditions. Any system that regulates the ebb and flow of fat into or out of fat storage depots must be able to sense and respond to fluctuations in our nutritional state in a flawless fashion. For example, we don't want to be in the fat-storing mode when we are starving because under such conditions we can die without food. In these circumstances we want to be able to burn all those stored calories to stay alive.

Because of its importance, a remarkably simple process has evolved that makes our energy storage system fail-safe. Or almost fail-safe, as we will see. When certain diseases derail it, we can lose weight effortlessly. On the other hand, when it gets stuck in the "on" position, we find ourselves gaining weight when we don't want to. To understand how it works, we need to "peer under the hood."

As we have seen, fat is stored in fat cells. When they get big, we get fat. As they shrink, we lose weight. To be successful, we need to know how to control the flow of fat into and out of these *temporary* fat storage depots. The key step in this entire process involves the cellular equivalent of a light switch that sits on the surface of each fat cell.

When viewed under a microscope, a fat cell looks like a balloon filled with yellow cheese. The balloon is the cell membrane —the coating that determines what is inside and outside the cell. Sitting on this cell membrane is a "switch" that can be flipped in one of two directions. When it is on, fat passes into the fat cell. When it is off, fat leaves the fat cell. Hormones play a key role in turning this fat-storing switch on and off.

Insulin—the Master Hormone

The ability to store fat has allowed the human race to survive for millions of years. However, no system is infallible. When things go awry, weight gain is one potential outcome. What we need to understand, however, is that to be beneficial, the handling of fat must be a two-way street. Fat must be able to enter fat cells when storage is appropriate and must also be able to exit when we need ready energy. Hormones are regulators of this delicate balance. They are the third link in the Brain–Belly connection.

As such, they control the flow of information about what we have eaten, what our energy requirements are, the status of our fat stores and the level of hunger. Immediately after we eat, there is abundant food energy available for the brain and the body. As the hours go by, we use up the food we have eaten and must be able to tap into our fat stores. For this to happen in a seamless fashion, the switch on fat cells must be thrown into the fat-releasing position as food energy is used up. Under these circumstances we don't get hungry because we rely on our *internal* source of calories —stored fat—as our energy source.

The hormone insulin controls the two-way switch that coordinates this process. It is the same hormone that regulates blood sugar levels, but is merely wearing a different hat—multitasking, if you will. When insulin is present at high levels, the switch is kept in the storage mode so that fat is collected, stored in fat cells and prevented from leaving. When insulin levels fall the switch snaps into the fat releasing position. This makes our stored fat available for use as an energy source to fuel our bodily processes. It also (appropriately) keeps us from getting hungry.

Fat is stored in fat cells. When they get big, we get fat. As they shrink, we lose weight. To be successful in losing weight, we need to know how to control the flow of fat into and out of these temporary fat storage depots.

What happens between meals after we have burned all the food calories we ate during our last meal (our external source of energy) if insulin levels remain elevated? High insulin generates a signal that keeps fat packed in fat cells and prevents it from being released for the body to use. Under these conditions our internal energy stores are not readily accessible, which causes our brain to respond by stimulating the appetite centers that send out hunger signals. So, as a result of being unable to burn stored fat, we end up eating more instead. This explains why losing weight is so difficult. *It is because the food we eat puts us in a persistent fat storing mode.* Overeating is the result!

As you can see, persistently elevated insulin levels prevent us from using our stored fat and make us hungry. We then eat more instead of doing what we want to do, which is burn stored fat. This is the worst position to be in for losing weight. In fact, it is the optimal scenario for gaining weight. Hence, the real villain here is insulin—specifically elevated insulin levels!

The Fat-Storing Trigger That Farmers Depend On

What has traditionally been the signal the body responds to when it is time to store calories as fat? Farmers know the answer all too well. Look at what they do in feedlots. They crowd animals together so they can't move around and expend energy (that is, exercise), and most importantly they feed them corn. As corn is digested it is converted into a type of sugar, which is a *potent signal for the release of insulin.* As a result of eating corn all day the animals' insulin levels remain elevated, which keeps them in a fat storing mode. They gain weight rapidly—just what the farmers want because they get paid by the pound. All the marbling in corn-fed beef is just this fat being stored in the meat.

This is a very effective method for making cattle bigger (actually fatter) because it increases fat storage (meaning fat going into fat cells) while simultaneously keeping the fat already in fat cells from being released. Our bodies work the same way. So, by

Persistently elevated insulin levels prevent us from using our stored fat and make us hungry.

eating corn and other similar foods that raise insulin levels, we get fat as well. Just think of it as "the feedlot syndrome."

If slimming your waistline doesn't give you sufficient motivation for cutting back on sugar consumption, consider the following results from a study done at the University of Alabama that demonstrated by reducing the intake of glucose (sugar) normal human cells age more slowly and the body is better able to weed out and eliminate precancerous cells.

Modern Fat Storage Signals—Better Than Anything Mother Nature Ever Devised

Carbohydrates like corn generate potent fat-storage signals because they cause insulin (the fat storage hormone) to remain elevated. However, not all carbohydrates are created equal. Insulin levels go up when blood glucose levels rise. Hence, foods that cause glucose levels to rise or remain high for too long are potent fat storage triggers because of their elevating impact on insulin levels.

Those foods that raise blood glucose levels more rapidly are the most effective at triggering insulin spikes (and fat storage). Vegetables and non-starchy fruits contain valuable nutrients and release their sugar slowly. They are important parts of any healthy diet. However, as man has cultivated and interbred various strains of foods, they have become more and more starchy. The luscious apples we see on our grocery shelves were not previously available. Apples that existed several hundred years ago were small and fibrous. They didn't taste very good because they didn't have the abundance of white sugar-filled fruit that we value today. They contained less "fruit" and more fiber—non-digestible carbohydrate.

What fruit sugar they did contain was released slowly, so it had very little impact on blood glucose (and subsequently insulin).

As a matter of fact, the most nutritious part of an apple is the red, green or yellow apple peel—something that is frequently removed and thrown away. This colorful rind provides a cornucopia of healthy antioxidants (free-radical fighters), anti-inflammatories and powerful phytonutrients.

Apples are obviously not the cause of the modern obesity trend. It is primarily the manufactured fat storage triggers that are to blame—industrially produced foods that fill our grocery shelves. They are much more effective at raising blood sugar levels than anything that ever existed naturally. Such foods are usually devoid of fiber and other nutrients, but are stuffed full of glucose molecules hooked end-to-end—a rapidly broken down and digested artificial food source that triggers insulin spikes more effectively than anything that preceded it.

They are the found in the so-called "packaged goods" section of the grocery store and include bread, cakes, crackers, candy, cookies, biscuits and sweetened beverages such as colas and fruit juices. Other bad actors that indirectly contribute to the development of obesity include table sugar (also called sucrose), high-fructose corn syrup (HFCS), crystalline fructose and all the foods that contain them. Believe me, they are in nearly everything so you need to read food labels carefully to weed them out. As an exercise, read the labels of items you would never expect to contain them such as ketchup or horseradish sauce.

Eating these foods keeps insulin levels elevated *long after a meal* and prevents fat from leaving fat cells to be used as an internal source of energy. When this happens, we get hungry too soon and eat more of the same foods—a process that is repeated multiple times each day. This leads to the creeping type of weight gain most of us experience around middle age—the real cause of the middle-aged middle.

Hence, it is the combination of an ancient evolutionarily based fat storage system (designed to save us during periods of starvation) that is being repeatedly triggered throughout the day (more potently than ever before) that has created the current obesity epidemic. Not only that, but, as we shall see, it has also created an epidemic of brain starvation.

Food Addicts!

It makes sense that fat storing machinery has become ingrained in our bodily chemistry, brain and genetic makeup because of the vital role it plays. However, consider for a moment the fact that the hunger and reward centers in the brain are close to each other and communicate freely. One implication of this proximity is that certain foods may interact with both simultaneously.

The reward system plays a key role in the addictive nature of drugs by reinforcing their use. The "high" that accompanies a heroin rush is both intensely pleasurable and of brief duration. For continued stimulation another "fix" is required. As a result the brain actually rewires itself to be on the lookout for whatever produced the "high." Alterations in nerve cells and how they are connected actually develop to facilitate the response—even to the point where it occurs subconsciously.

The same reaction can be fostered when we eat. Comfort foods are the prime offenders. They have potentially addictive properties because they make us feel good. As a result, we look forward to the next sweet, savory bite. A pleasure response is generated and is repeatedly reinforced. Food manufacturers understand this addiction all too well—the universe of such food products on the market today is testimony to that fact.

Food additives and sweeteners are able to augment the addictive properties of food. As an example, on the sweetness rating scale glucose (the primary "sugar" in blood) weighs in at a measly 0.8. Compare that with table sugar (sucrose) that is rated

1.0. High fructose corn syrup is 1.2. And fructose is 1.4—almost twice as sweet as glucose.

Where do artificial sweeteners fall on this same scale? Aspartame is listed at 180, acesulfame at 200 and saccharin (Sweet'N Low) at 300, while sucralose (Splenda) weighs in at 600. This means Splenda is 750 times as sweet as glucose! No wonder so many of us are addicted to foods containing these super sweet additives.

• • •

As we have seen, being able to store food energy as fat has enabled us to survive repeated famines. Animals that don't have this ability live short lives. However, living successfully without storing *excess* fat means that we must use our fat cells as they were intended to be used—as temporary food energy reservoirs, not permanent and expanding fat stores. The key to success is knowing what food choices to make to keep fat cells functioning as two-way streets.

2
The Clamor of Hunger—
Lessons from Five Diets

You learned in Chapter 1 that eating foods that raise your insulin level quickly, and keep it elevated, prevents your body from getting rid of fat. We're also frequently told that we eat too much and don't exercise enough. So you'll be very interested to hear that similar factors help determine when you get hungry—and how hungry you feel.

It seems logical to assume that if you don't eat enough food you'll get the munchies and if you eat too much you won't. However, numerous studies have shown that this assumption is not always true—or at least that the correlation between how much you eat and how hungry you feel is not as direct as it might seem. Most of us have had similar personal experiences so this should come as no surprise. Studying the way our bodies react to how much we eat—and *what* we eat—can help us to understand the right way to eat so we don't feel hungry all the time.

Let's examine five different "diets"—some producing seemingly paradoxical results—and see what they teach us.

Five Diets

1. Calorie-Restricted Low Fat Diet

In one study that investigated this type of diet, twelve healthy young men of normal weight ate 1,400 to 2,100 calories per day (the usual caloric intake for them would have been about 3,000–3,200 calories per day) with the intent of lowering their body weight by about 10 percent in a month. The stated purpose of the study was to see if humans could "adjust to this lower nutritional level and thrive."

Result: *The desired weight loss occurred, but the men were constantly hungry and felt cold.*

In 1944 Ancil Keys performed a similar experiment over a longer period of time. His subjects were overweight men who were restricted to 1,570 calories per day—about one-half of what had been required for them to maintain their weight previously. The diet consisted primarily of "whole-wheat bread, potatoes, cereals, and considerable amounts of turnips and cabbage." The composition was 57.3 percent carbohydrate (about 900 calories), 17.2 percent fat (about 270 calories), and 25.4 percent protein (about 400 calories)—a macronutrient breakdown that resembles diets that many people follow today.

One of Keys's goals was to document the psychological response to severe (about 50 percent) caloric restriction on a low fat diet. He reported that the participants complained of unremitting and ravenous hunger. Food became a preoccupation. Plates and silverware were licked clean. The mere act of waiting in line to be served was frequently overwhelming, and neuroses and psychoses were not uncommon. Subjects also complained of always feeling cold.

While this diet may appear excessively severe, its calorie restriction is within the realm of what are considered conventional reducing diets today—with similar results—persistent hunger!

2. Calorie-Restricted Higher-Fat Diet

In 1936 Per Hanssen published a report that suggested that *nutrient content in addition to caloric content* might be vital in determining how the body responds to dietary changes. He treated twenty-one obese subjects with an 1850-calorie diet composed of

25 percent carbohydrate (about 470 calories), 60 percent fat (about 1,100 calories) and 15 percent protein (about 280 calories). It is interesting to note that Hanssen's diet contained four times the fat content used by Ancil Keys.

Result: Hanssen's subjects stayed on the diet from one to four months, lost an average of two pounds per week and never felt hungry even while eating **approximately the same number of calories** *as were consumed on the Keys diet.*

3. Total Starvation Diet

On a total starvation diet (such as the example discussed at the beginning of Chapter 1 describing the plane crash survivors Helen Klaben and Ralph Flores), subjects drink water but eat no food at all. On this type of diet, all of the calories burned are those that are released from body stores. After a few days of not eating approximately 70 percent of the calories burned are from fat cells and the remaining 30 percent are from muscle breakdown and glucose. Under these circumstances if the carbohydrate contribution (glucose) is about 20 percent, the fat-to-carb calorie ratio in the nutrients being utilized is 3.5:1 (70:20).

Result: After a few days of starvation, subjects' hunger abates, food cravings disappear and weight is lost!

4. Cruise Ship Diet

If you've ever taken a cruise, you've undoubtedly been stunned by the amount of food you eat—a sumptuous breakfast, large lunch, pizza at 3 PM, frequent snacks, dessert extravaganzas and midnight feeds—often with your only physical activity consisting of lounging around the pool while sipping island punch.

> *It is interesting to note that Hanssen's diet contained four times the fat content of Keys' diet.*

Result: In such situations, most people find themselves getting hungry despite the large number of calories they're taking in—and, not surprisingly, gaining weight.

5. Typical American Diet

It may surprise you to learn that the dietary composition (meaning the relative contributions of protein, fat and carbohydrate) of many Americans is not too different from the first diet we looked at—the low fat diet—but with more calories and often containing lots of rapidly digested carbohydrates and very few healthy fats, proteins, or fiber.

Result: The typical American on this "typical" diet is likely to be overweight.

Let's Compare

This table summarizes some information about the diets just described.

NAME OF DIET	CALORIES	CARBO-HYDRATE	FAT	PROTEIN	FAT:CARB RATIO	RESULT
1 Keys Low-Fat Diet	1,570 (Low calorie diet)	57.3% (900 calories)	17.2% (270 calories)	25.4% (400 calories)	0.3:1	Weight loss; constant hunger; feeling cold
2 Hanssen Higher Fat Diet	1,850 (Low calorie diet)	25% (470 calories)	60% (1,100 calories)	15% (280 calories)	2.4:1	Weight loss; no hunger
3 Total Starvation	0 (No calorie diet)	20% (from internal stores)	70% (from internal stores)	10% (from internal stores)	3.5:1	Weight loss; no hunger
4 Cruise Ship Diet	4,500 (High calorie diet)	50% (2,250 calories)	30% (1,350 calories)	20% (900 calories)	0.6:1	Weight gain; frequent hunger
5 Typical American Diet	2,500 ("Typical" diet)	55% (1,375 calories)	30% (750 calories)	15% (375 calories)	0.55:1	Weight gain; frequent hunger

Some Important Concepts

Before you learn how these very different diets can produce the seemingly paradoxical results they do, it's helpful to be aware of some important concepts: *metabolic rate, internal versus external sources of energy* and *nutrients versus calories.*

Feel Cold? Check Your Metabolic Rate

Most subjects on fairly severely calorie-restricted diets find that they are constantly cold even when dressed warmly. Humans are warm-blooded animals, which means that they must keep their metabolic rate (the amount of energy the body uses in a given period) high enough to stay warm and keep the body's biochemical reactions humming along at the correct rate.

When your brain thinks you're starving, one of its first responses is to lower your *metabolic rate* in order to reduce your caloric requirements. The idea is that if you use less energy, you'll need fewer calories, which is a good thing if food is scarce. But having a low metabolic rate also makes you feel cold.

Notice that I said when your brain *thinks* you're starving. We'll find out that sometimes your brain *thinks* you're starving when you're not!

Food versus Stored Fat:
External versus Internal Sources of Energy

The food you eat is your *external* source of energy. Your stored fat—what I like to call your *built-in pantries*—is your *internal* source of energy. Your brain can tell your body when to use this internal source, or—by making you feel hungry—when you need to use an external source (meaning eat more). Sometimes, however, even though your built-in pantries contain ample energy, your body is unable to access that energy and, as a result, your brain senses a lack of nutrition and makes you feel hungry. So you eat more food rather than rely on your fat stores—not what you want to do if losing weight is your goal.

A Calorie Is a Calorie, Right? Nutrients versus Calories

If you compare the number of calories in the Keys and Hanssen diets, you'll see that they're similar: 1,570 and 1,850. However, if you compare the *nutrients* in the two diets, you'll notice a huge difference in the ratio of fats to carbohydrates. As you can see in the table below, the Hanssen diet contains about four times as much fat and eight times as many fat calories *per carbohydrate calorie* as the Keys diet (2.4 versus 0.3).

NAME OF DIET	FAT CALORIES	CARBOHYDRATE CALORIES	APPROXIMATE RATIO OF FATS TO CARBOHYDRATES	HUNGRY?
Keys	17.2% (270 calories)	57.3% (900 calories)	0.3:1 (0.3 calories of fat for each calorie of carbohydrate)	Yes
Hanssen	60% (1,100 calories	25% (470 calories)	2.4:1 (2.4 calories of fat for each calorie of carbohydrate)	No

The subjects on the Ancil Keys diet were hungry all the time and those on the Per Hanssen diet were not. What about the Cruise Ship diet and the Starvation diet? You would think that eating many more calories than your body requires would suppress appetite while eating no calories would make you hungry. So why does the opposite happen? Let's compare the ratios of fats to carbohydrates and see what they suggest.

NAME OF DIET	FAT CALORIES	CARBOHYDRATE CALORIES	APPROXIMATE RATIO OF FATS TO CARBOHYDRATES	HUNGRY?
Cruise Ship	30% (1,350 calories)	50% (2,250 calories)	0.6:1 (0.6 calories of fat for each calorie of carbohydrate)	Yes
Starvation (calories burned are from internal sources)	70%	20%	3.5:1 (3.5 calories of fat for each calorie of carbohydrate)	No

On the Cruise Ship diet appetite increases in spite of eating excessive numbers of calories. However, during a brief period of total starvation, appetite falls. This doesn't seem to make sense from the perspective of caloric intake. Just the opposite would be expected—the people eating nothing should be hungrier than those aboard the cruise liner who shouldn't be hungry at all.

However, could the nutrient content of the diet suggest an explanation? Hanssen's diet contained a high fat-to-carbohydrate ratio (2.4:1) that resembles the much higher starvation ratio of 3.5:1. Both of these seemed to be associated with less hunger. The Cruise Ship and Keys diets had low ratios (0.3:1 and 0.6:1, respectively) and the subjects on them were hungrier.

This observation suggests that the *kind* of calories you eat as well as the total number of calories consumed might make a difference in how your body responds to them and must be taken into consideration. A diet with a higher (and healthier) fat intake and a greater fat to carb ratio appears to be much more effective at producing satiety. Since you eat more when you are hungry, it seems as if the type of food that is consumed—in addition to its calorie content—makes a large difference in what you weigh.

In the next chapter I will try to shed some light on why this might be the case.

3
Controlling Your Appetite
by Feeding Your Brain

You might be wondering what the connection is between feeding your brain and controlling your appetite. Well, whether you are daydreaming about a certain food, feeling hungry or just plain wanting to nosh—these are all brain states. There is an intimate connection between the brain, food and the way we think about it. After all, from the brain's perspective, the body—including its ability to ambulate—is just a sophisticated conveyance designed to deliver food to the brain. Its appetite centers are merely the mechanism for making its feelings about food known.

You have probably noticed when you are hungry it is not uncommon to have difficulty concentrating. When neurons in the appetite centers sense a lack of nutrients, they send out a hunger signal. Under similar conditions neurons in other regions of the brain react as well. However, since they mediate different functions such as focus and concentration, when they suffer from brain starvation symptoms like brain fog or mental fatigue appear. However, in both circumstances the cause is identical—the brain has not been fed properly.

What Happens When You Eat?

There are two basic fuels that your body depends on for energy—carbohydrates (foods that are broken down into glucose) and fat. Depending upon what you have eaten, and when, the fuel mixture your body burns at any point in time consists of a combination of both fat and glucose. However, the amount each contributes varies dramatically throughout the day. Right after a meal, glucose is the primary fuel. In between meals or while you are fasting—such as at night when you are asleep—the fuel mix contains a much higher fat content.

Also, when one fuel contributes more to the mixture being burned the other plays a lesser role. So, they both go through reciprocal peaks and valleys during a 24-hour cycle. It sounds complicated, but the basics are pretty easy to understand.

As you learned in Chapter 1, when you eat your blood glucose (blood "sugar") level rises and nourishes your body and brain. The presence of glucose in the blood also causes the insulin level to increase. Insulin controls blood sugar by transporting it out of the blood and into the cells of the body where it is burned up. This is why glucose is the primary source of energy when the insulin level rises after a meal.

At the same time, when insulin is high fat gets sent into fat cells *for storage*—to be released after the carbohydrates that have just been eaten are used up. So, the rise and fall of insulin causes the fuel mixture to fluctuate between sugar and fat. High insulin (which occurs after a meal) triggers fat storage and sugar burning. In between meals, when insulin is low, fat is released for use as a fuel source. If everything is in synch these nutrients move back and forth providing the energy we need exactly when it is required. It's just that at certain times energy is generated from sugar while at other times fat is the primary fuel source.

Although every meal we consume has a different fat and carbohydrate composition, a similar overall response occurs each time we eat. Glucose is burned first while insulin is storing the fat that will be made available for use after the glucose is gone. It is the waxing and waning of the hormone insulin that coordinates this delicate process.

What *should* happen once the glucose and fat from the prior meal have been completely burned is that you start feeling hungry again. However, things don't always work as they are supposed to. To see what I mean let's look at an example of what happens to two people, John and Jane, after breakfast and how making the wrong food choices can produce disastrous results.

An Ideal Scenario: John's Morning

John starts to eat breakfast at 8:00. From shortly after 8:00 until about 9:30 his blood sugar level rises. This (appropriately) causes his insulin level to rise, which starts sugar burning while sending fat to be stored in his fat cells (his built-in pantries). By about 10:30 he has used up the initial rush of food energy from breakfast, his insulin level has decreased and his fat cells release their stored energy for use as fuel for another couple of hours. Around noon after both the initial food energy and the stored fat that was released are gone, he starts to feel hungry again.

Let's look at a graph of the changes that occurred in John's body after breakfast. In Figure 3.1 you will see two curves—one that depicts his glucose level (solid black) and one that charts his insulin level (dashed). During the interval depicted by the letter "A" he is in a fat-burning mode that started while he was sleeping the prior evening when his insulin level was low. As his glucose and insulin levels begin to go up after breakfast (see the letter "B"), he starts burning glucose and simultaneously enters the fat-storing zone. This happens because his increasing insulin level activates the fat storing switches on his fat cells.

At about 10:30, shown by the letter "C," his glucose and insulin levels have fallen which allow his fat cells to start releasing fat to burn for energy. It becomes the fuel source that carries him to lunchtime when he becomes hungry again.

That's the ideal situation. However, as we saw in Chapter 2, apparently not all calories are treated equally. To see what I mean, let's look at Jane's morning.

When insulin is high fat gets sent into fat cells for storage.

Figure 3.1: John's Morning

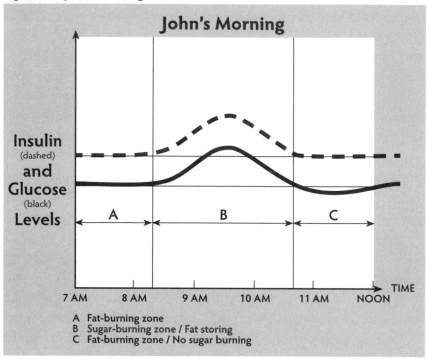

A   Fat-burning zone
B   Sugar-burning zone / Fat storing
C   Fat-burning zone / No sugar burning

A Not-So-Ideal Scenario: Jane's Morning

Jane also began eating breakfast at 8:00. She and John are about the same size and eat the same number of calories. From 8:00 to 10:30 she used some of the energy from the food she ate while an increasing insulin level directed her body to store the rest of it in her fat cells. So far it sounds just like John's morning. But at about 10:30 Jane started feeling hungry again.

Let's examine the graph (see Figure 3.2) and see what happened to her after breakfast. As shown by the letter "D" she began the day in a fat-burning mode that started the previous evening. After breakfast, because of the rise in insulin she entered the sugar-burning and fat-storing mode (as John did) depicted by the letter "E." This continued until about 10:30 when, like John (see "F"), she

Figure 3.2: Jane's Morning

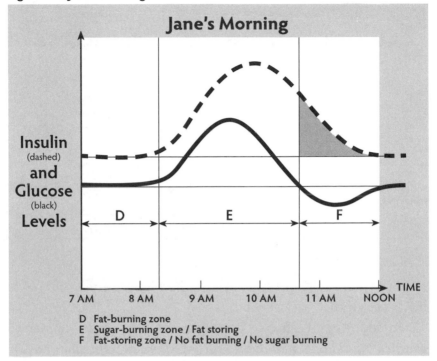

left the sugar burning zone. However, because of her persistently elevated insulin level (see the dashed insulin curve that is still elevated at 10:30) she was *still in the fat-storing mode* (see the shaded area under the insulin curve from 10:30 to noon). This is when she began to feel hungry. What made her appetite suddenly increase at 10:30 even though she ate the same number of calories as John?

What's the Difference between These Two Scenarios?

Comparing Figures 3.1 and 3.2 you can see that by about 10:30 the glucose level for both John and Jane has fallen back to its baseline value. The noticeable difference in the figures is that Jane's glucose curve peaked at a higher level than John's and she

Table 3.1

JOHN'S BREAKFAST DESCRIPTION (EATEN AS A MIXTURE)	CALORIES	CARB CAL.	FAT CAL.	PROTEIN CAL.	FAT TO CARB CALORIE RATIO
½ cup of strawberries	25	21	0	4	
½ cup blueberries	42	38	1	3	
¾ cup cottage cheese	180	28	70	82	
¼ cup regular plain yogurt	38	12	18	8	
⅛ cup sliced almonds	68	4	51	13	
½ Tbsp flax seed oil	60	0	60	0	
¼ tsp ground cinnamon	0	0	0	0	
Total	**413**	**103** (25%)	**200** (48%)	**110** (27%)	**1.9:1**

required more insulin (as shown by the higher insulin curve) to bring her glucose back down.

In addition, because of her higher glucose peak *she had an elevated insulin level that didn't return to normal until almost noon.* (Compare her insulin level to John's.) It remained high *even after her blood sugar level returned to normal.* This persistently elevated insulin level kept her in a fat-storing mode for an extra ninety minutes (depicted by the shaded area under her insulin curve from 10:30 to 12:00). In contrast, John was back in a fat-burning mode again by 10:30 (when his insulin level had come back to normal).

Jane, however, was prevented from tapping into her fat stores when she needed them at 10:30. Since she had essentially no access to fat or glucose from 10:30 on, she got hungry before John did. But the important question is—why did this happen?

Let's examine what each of them ate for breakfast. (See Tables 3.1 and 3.2.) As you can see, the number of calories were identical —413. However, John's ratio of fat to carbohydrate calories was 1.9:1, while Jane's was much lower at 0.23:1—meaning that he

Table 3.2

JANE'S BREAKFAST DESCRIPTION	CALORIES	CARB CAL.	FAT CAL.	PROTEIN CAL.	FAT TO CARB CALORIE RATIO
1 cup corn flakes	100	91	0	9	
½ cup 2% fat milk	62	16	22	24	
1 cup orange juice	110	103	0	7	
1 slice whole wheat toast	65	40	9	16	
1 pat butter	36	0	36	0	
½ ounce grape jelly	40	40	0	0	
Total	**413**	**290** (70%)	**67** (16%)	**56** (14%)	**0.23:1**

ate more fat and less carbohydrate than she did. Since fat calories impact glucose and insulin levels minimally, it is no surprise that John's glucose and insulin levels were much lower than Jane's.

In addition, the *type* of carbohydrates Jane chose to eat contained less fiber. By slowing down absorption fiber blunts the rate at which glucose levels rise and subsequently prevents high insulin levels from developing. The presence of fiber in food is what makes it a slow release form of carbohydrate. Hence, the fiberless carbs she ate for breakfast were more rapidly absorbed and produced higher glucose and insulin levels.

Since her high insulin level kept fat locked in fat cells and thus prevented her from using it as fuel when she needed it, her appetite increased. This was why Jane got hungry much sooner than John did.

When the brain doesn't receive the nutrients it requires to function properly, something I call brain starvation, it generates a hunger signal. If it is properly nourished it functions flawlessly and hunger doesn't develop. This is the critical link between food, brains and appetite. So, *what* we eat can be as important as *how much* we eat because of how it affects the way the food calories are handled by the body—meaning whether they end up being stored or burned!

Foods that stimulate this type of hormonal response (a rapid and sustained rise in insulin) make the body think it is starving when that is not the case at all. In fact, most of us have plenty of stored fat—sometimes enough to last for several months. The problem is that it can't be released because the fat storage switch can't be turned off. This is precisely what happened to Jane and why she got hungry prematurely and had to eat again at 10:30.

I have chosen a man and woman (John and Jane) to illustrate how what we eat is as important as how many calories we consume. The outcome would have been the same if two men or two women had been used in this example.

Foods That *Fool* Your Body

Jane got hungry *as a result of prolonged, excessive and unwanted fat storage.* This happened because of the food choices she made during breakfast. As you can see in Figure 3.2, when she needed to switch from using sugar to fat her high insulin level prevented her from doing so.

She became hungry *even before her body had used up what she had just eaten!* So, by making the wrong food choices she was "tricked" into eating again when she shouldn't have been hungry at all! *And it had nothing to do with the number of calories she ate.* She simply made food choices that produced signals that were interpreted by her brain as hunger because of how the food was handled internally—that is, it went into a storage rather than a delivery form.

It is no surprise that we can't survive without food. But because we have the ability to store food for use between meals, we don't have to eat continuously. Hormones are the chemical conductors that orchestrate the delicate process that determines how the energy from food is used. When they are in proper balance,

Hormones are the chemical conductors that orchestrate the delicate process that determines how the energy from food is used.

the ebb and flow of nutrients are carefully regulated to provide a continual supply of energy that exactly matches our metabolic requirements. We are not prevented from running or being active simply because we haven't eaten and, likewise, we won't get hungry between meals.

When hormones are doing their job properly, all is well. But how they work depends on the types of food choices we make. The interaction between food and hormones is an ancient one dating back millions of years. It evolved based on the body's responses to foods that were present during that same period.

However, in recent times eating habits have changed dramatically. About eighty percent of the food on the shelves of supermarkets today didn't exist 100 years ago. Much of it is "manufactured" food that has been produced in factories rather than having been derived more directly from plants or animals.

To understand how this difference affects the body let's look at what Jane ate for breakfast. Several foods—especially the corn flakes, OJ, toast and jelly—triggered a large, prolonged surge of insulin because of the rapidly released carbohydrates they contain. This hormonal response was necessary to properly regulate Jane's blood glucose level. However, it takes the body a long time to bring such a high insulin level back down to normal. This excessive insulin surge keeps fat sequestered in fat cells at a time when the calories contained within them are needed to fuel the body. The result is a nutrient shortfall that is interpreted by the brain as impending starvation. This example illustrates how poor food choices can trick us into eating when our "pantries" may be bursting with stored calories.

She Eats Like a Bird and Still Gains Weight!

Can this really happen? And if so, how can it possibly be explained? Let's see if we can make sense of this scenario using some of the principles we have just discussed.

As we already know, appetite increases when the brain senses an impending food shortage. The same thing happens when insulin levels remain high and prevent us from accessing the fat stored in our pantries. One occurs because of a shortage of "external" calories (food) and the other from a shortage of "internal" calories (being unable to access stored fat).

If either of these conditions persists the brain responds by slowing down the rate at which calories are burned (also referred to as metabolic rate or metabolism). This is how the body goes into "starvation mode," which is a response that allows it to survive longer using its fat stores. It was this process that allowed Helen Klaben and Ralph Flores to successfully endure their harrowing plane crash discussed in Chapter 1. However, while a slower metabolism allows us to survive for a longer time when we are starving, it also means that it takes longer to burn fat and lose weight while dieting.

We are all familiar with people who ostensibly eat very few calories, are hungry all the time and in spite of this, gain weight. Whenever I was confronted with this scenario in the past I found it difficult to believe. As a matter of fact, my initial reaction was that they were eating much more than they thought and that was the logical explanation for their weight gain.

We now have the tools to postulate another mechanism to explain how it might happen. Imagine someone eating a reduced calorie diet to lose weight. At first the pounds come off. Then a weight loss plateau frequently occurs. One explanation for this is that the metabolic rate has slowed down and the number of calories being consumed just matches the number being burned— now a smaller number per day because of the slower metabolism.

To start the weight loss process again, even fewer calories are consumed. After a while metabolism slows further and weight loss again sputters. The cycle must be repeated again with even fewer calories. This is frequently how bird-like diets are initiated.

Now consider being on this type of diet and, in addition, including mostly foods that repeatedly spike insulin levels. These are bread, cookies, soda pop and other comfort-type foods that will cause the calories being consumed to go directly to fat cells where they are stored rather than being burned (because of the insulin spikes). In this example, if the number of calories being consumed is about 1,200 and 400 of them end up being locked in fat cells, it is really equivalent to eating only 800 calories since that is what the body has available to use.

That is truly eating like a bird—a starving bird. Under these circumstances metabolism slows drastically, possibly to the point where the body is only burning 700 calories in a twenty four hour period. This would mean that 100 calories are being stored each day (the difference between 800 and 700)—a situation in which weight is being gained while eating like a bird!

Hence, by restricting calories and making the wrong food choices two things happen—*metabolism slows* and we *starve internally* (by storing calories in fat cells where they are locked up and become inaccessible). Together, these conspire to enable us to store fat, gain weight, feel constantly hungry and do so on a starvation diet!

Appetite increases when insulin levels remain high and prevent us from accessing the fat stored in our pantries.

How is this situation to be avoided? First, don't cut calories. This merely serves as a signal for metabolism to slow. Second, prevent the body from sending what you eat to fat cells for storage. The way to achieve this is by choosing foods that keep insulin levels low—slow-release carbohydrates, protein and healthy fats. When you do this your body makes the transition from burning external calories to burning internal calories— your fat stores. Under these circumstances metabolism doesn't slow down, hunger doesn't develop and fat cells shrink. This is what must be accomplished if weight loss is to be achieved.

If you know someone in this situation, do them a favor and tell them what to do about it!

A Multi-Tasking Hormone

What you eat determines your blood glucose level, which, in turn, is responsible for telling the body how much insulin is required at any specific point in time. However, a problem arises after the consumption of large amounts of refined carbohydrates because the excessively high insulin level that is required to process the onslaught of glucose eventually stimulates one's appetite centers. The ultimate source of the glucose in the bloodstream is the carbohydrate content in the diet. None of it comes from the fat and protein we eat. This demonstrates how our food choices directly determine insulin levels, and subsequently, appetite and fat storage.

In addition to being the hormone that controls blood sugar levels, insulin is also the *fat storage* hormone. The ability to wear both of these metabolic hats makes the hormonal system more efficient, but at the same time *ties the glucose-regulating and fat-storing systems together*. This has very important implications for knowing what to eat to stay thin. When we examined the different effects of what John and Jane ate for breakfast, you saw what impact their food choices had in real life.

The more carbohydrates you eat, the higher your insulin will go—and high is not good if you want to stay thin or lose weight. However, not all carbs are created equal. Those that are rapidly digested are the worst offenders and include most packaged goods such as cakes, cereals, cookies, crackers, candy, chips, snack foods, sugary beverages, breads, rolls, donuts and pastries. Also included are starchy foods such as potatoes and rice. The "good" carbs (those that are very slowly broken down and absorbed over hours—thus acting as a slowly released form of carbohydrate) are usually the non-starchy fruits and vegetables including salad greens, berries, asparagus, broccoli, peppers, chard, kale, and their neighbors on the grocery store shelves.

You may have heard that "complex" carbs are the healthy ones. This is not always the case. Consider, for example, bread or potatoes. They contain complex carbs but in a form that is rapidly released. Most "good" carbs are combined with fiber. The body very slowly absorbs this form of complex carbohydrate because the fiber acts like glue that slows down the release of the attached sugar into the bloodstream.

As you can see, when your insulin level is high, your body is in fat-storage mode. When it's low, your body is primed to burn fat. If your insulin level stays high most of the time, your body is nearly always in *fat storage* mode and hardly ever has a chance to release its stored fat for the body to use. This is what causes you to gain weight. It is your food choices that directly control *how hard your body wants to hang onto fat*—and subsequently, how likely you are to gain weight. If you feel that fat just seems to stick to your body like glue, this is the reason why.

> *The more carbohydrates you eat, the higher your insulin will go—and high is not good if you want to stay thin or lose weight.*

"Sticky" Fat Cells

The amount of fat in your fat cells is determined not just by how much fat *enters* them, but also by how much fat *leaves* them. When the amount entering and the amount leaving over a period of time are equal, fat cells don't enlarge. They properly perform their job of storing fat *temporarily* as you eat and releasing it between meals so that you don't feel hungry before your next meal. You can see that when they're used in this way, fat cells are not intrinsically evil. In fact, they serve a very useful purpose—they allow you to do important tasks such as go to work, pick up the kids or relax instead of having to eat constantly to maintain your energy level.

However, if poor food choices are made problems arise because healthy fat cells become what I call "sticky"—meaning they accumulate calories when you eat, but don't release them between meals. As a result, fat cells keep enlarging and you gain weight. How does this happen?

Insulin: The Operator of Your Fat Cells' On-Off Switch

As with many other similar biological processes, a cellular "switch" is involved. When it is on, your fat cells act like magnets and collect every speck of fat they encounter. When it is off, the cells release fat. It turns out that insulin is intimately involved in this on-off process. When your insulin level is high, it turns the switch on and your fat cells are locked in the fat-storing mode. In this situation they are unable to release their stored fat. When your insulin level is low, the switch is turned off, and fat can be released for use by the body.

What happens if your insulin level stays high most of the time? When this happens your fat cells stay locked in storage mode, and they keep getting larger and larger. Not only that, but because the energy in that stored fat is not available to be properly used, nutrient levels fall and your brain's appetite centers tell you it's time to eat again.

So as you can see, you don't get fat because you *eat* too many calories, but because you've *stored*—and continue to store—too many calories as fat and *can't access that fat between meals*. You're providing your brain and body with enough energy, but you're storing an excess amount of fat while doing so. For this reason I call gaining weight a *fat storage problem*. To see what I mean, look at the banking analogy on the next page.

She Stored Too Much Fat, So She Overate

As we have seen, John and Jane ate the same number of calories for breakfast. However, Jane got hungry long before John did. This happened because of the types of foods she chose to eat. The hormonal response they generated caused her fat cells to become sticky and she got hungry much earlier than John— in spite of eating an identical number of calories! The sticky fat cells stored fat (so far, so good), but later after she had used up the initial surge of energy from breakfast and had to rely on the energy locked away in her fat cells, they weren't able to release it. This energy shortfall was sensed by her brain, which then stimulated her appetite centers causing her to overeat. If this scenario is repeated throughout the day, weight gain is inevitable because she will store excess fat, get hungry, overeat and repeat the process again and again.

As shown in Figure 3.2, by about 10:30 Jane had used up the glucose from breakfast, but because her insulin level was still high she couldn't access the fat she had just stored and got hungry as a result. Thus, in spite of eating the same number of calories as John did, she got hungry and he didn't because of the high insulin level her breakfast choices produced, and the sticky fat cells that developed.

So, the take-home message is that Jane overate because she stored too much fat. She didn't get fat because she ate too much. This is an important distinction because if she gained weight as the

· ·

Banking Analogy

Suppose you have a job that pays you $1,000 every Friday. And every Friday you deposit $300 in a savings account and keep $700 to spend for rent, food, gas and so forth. Over the weekend, the bank is closed and you can't withdraw money from your savings account so, in effect, that $300 doesn't exist—it's as if you were paid only $700.

The $300 in your savings account is like the calories you store in your fat cells, which are also unavailable for you to use for energy. The difference is that on Monday you'll be able to withdraw your $300, whereas unless you start eating differently, the calories in your fat cells are permanently locked up!

· ·

result of overeating, then the correct solution would be to eat less. However, she ate too much because she developed sticky fat cells. In this case, *the appropriate response is to make proper food choices that prevent sticky fat cells from developing—not to eat less!* Nonstick fat cells will then, in turn, prevent you from overeating.

Now, armed with this knowledge we can tackle the diet paradoxes from Chapter 2.

Making Sense of the Diet Paradoxes

In the previous chapter I described five diets—two low-calorie diets that produced opposite results, a starvation diet that suppressed appetite, a gluttonous diet that increased appetite and a "typical" American diet. Let's see how what we've learned about insulin and its effect on fat cells explains these almost counterintuitive results.

The Keys Experiment

In the Keys experiment overweight, healthy subjects were forced to eat a diet that was low in calories and low in fat. They lost weight but were cold and hungry all the time. The type of carbohydrates they ate kept their insulin level high (making their fat cells sticky in the process). This made their fat stores inaccessible. That plus the fact that they were eating only about half the calories they usually did made them feel ravenously hungry. Eating less food slowed their metabolism and made them feel cold. Ironically, obese people (with even bigger "pantries") who follow similar diets also get hungry. Because their fat cells are sticky they can't tap into the large amount of stored fat they carry around.

The Hanssen Experiment

The Hanssen subjects ate about the same number of calories as the Keys subjects but they didn't feel hungry. Why? Because they were eating food with a higher fat content that didn't substantially raise their insulin levels. As a result, their fat cells were able to release stored energy that prevented them from getting hungry and allowed them to lose weight in the process.

Total Starvation

When subjects eat no food at all, insulin levels plummet. Their fat cells become "un-sticky" and are able to release stored fat thus providing all of the calories the brain and body need. So, in spite of eating no calories, no hunger develops.

Cruise Ship Eating

How can cruise ship guests eat so much and still be hungry all the time? The food they eat generates extremely high and persistently elevated insulin levels that keep their fat cells sticky. Consequently, a couple of hours after eating they feel hungry, eat again and repeat this process over and over. So, in spite of eating many thousands of calories each day, they actually are hungrier than if they hadn't eaten anything at all.

The Typical American Diet

The typical American diet, which is filled with starchy vegetables (like french fries) and processed foods as well as sugar-laden drinks, keeps insulin levels and hunger levels high much as the Keys diet did. You can see the result wherever you go in the United States—a shocking number of obese adults and children.

Diabetes: How Does It Help to Explain Insulin's Role in Fat Storage and Weight Gain?

If I haven't convinced you of the importance of controlling your insulin levels, here's something else to think about. What happens when, because of a disease (diabetes), someone's body doesn't produce any insulin?

Jay Cutler's Secret

The following anecdote will give you an important perspective about the impact of insulin on body weight.

In 2007 Jay Cutler was the quarterback for the Denver Broncos football team. It is no secret that you have to be big and strong to survive in professional sports. However, during the course of that season he lost almost 35 pounds. *This occurred despite training with weights, regularly eating thousands of calories per day and taking numerous nutritional supplements.*

How could this happen? The short answer is that although he was 24 he developed a childhood disease—diabetes mellitus (Type 1 diabetes)—a condition in which an inflammatory process destroyed the cells in his pancreas, the organ that makes insulin. Childhood diabetes usually develops this way. Jay Cutler just happened to be a young adult when his body was attacked. Without any insulin to store energy (meaning fat, glucose and protein), he lost almost 15 percent of his body mass *even though he was doing everything he could to gain weight.* This observation will help you understand how to lose weight easily.

Why did this happen and how does it relate to our current dietary discussion? As Jay Cutler learned, when your body can't produce much insulin weight loss occurs very rapidly—*in spite of eating a large number of calories.* Why? To gain weight there must be a signal telling the body to *store* the energy provided by the calories you eat. Otherwise they will be burned up. Insulin is just that signal. A diet that produces a high insulin signal directs the body to store fat, and a diet that minimizes the food storage signal (by keeping insulin levels low) usually produces weight loss.

Juvenile diabetes (a disease that destroys the body's ability to produce insulin) is merely an extreme example of this phenomenon. People who develop juvenile diabetes usually make *no* insulin, and as a result, they lose weight—a lot of weight. This is so consistent a response that it is one of the first symptoms doctors look for when they see a child who might be developing juvenile diabetes.

What about Adult-Onset (Type 2) Diabetes?

It is important to understand the fundamental distinction between what happens in juvenile diabetes and what typically occurs in Type 2 diabetes (usually seen in overweight people). In adults who are on the road to developing Type 2 diabetes, insulin levels are frequently quite high—much higher than normal—because of poor dietary choices. They stay elevated until the pancreas can't keep up with the demands placed on it. When this happens, adult onset diabetes develops.

Type 2 diabetics are usually overweight or obese and have elevated insulin levels. However, even though their insulin levels are elevated, they aren't able to produce enough insulin to regulate their blood sugar, so they need even more. This is why Type 2 diabetics often require insulin injections—to augment what their body is producing. *However, when adult diabetics are put on insulin therapy they usually gain weight, just as Jay Cutler did after he started insulin injections.*

It All Adds Up!

By doing a little math, let's see how avoiding sticky fat cells can make a huge difference. For example, consider a typical healthy male who is 5'10" and weighs 150 pounds when he graduates from college at age 22. Assume that he eats three meals and one snack a day. According to the USDA (U.S. Department of Agriculture) Economic Research Service (last updated 12/21/2004), the *average* American consumes 120 pounds of sugar/HFCS (high-fructose corn syrup) per year. That averages out to be about 150 grams (almost one third of a pound!) per day, or a little less than 40 grams per meal for our "typical" subject.

This alone is sufficient to produce four fat-storing periods a day. If each contributes merely one gram of stored fat per meal, it adds up to four grams of fat storage per day. This is equivalent to 36 stored calories per day, or almost four pounds per year. What that means for this unlucky fellow is that by the time he reaches his 32nd birthday he will weigh not 150 pounds (his weight at graduation) but an astounding 190 pounds! In just ten more years he will weigh in at a portly 230 pounds as he hits middle age.

A quote attributed to Albert Einstein, the father of the modern theory of gravity, stated, "The most powerful force in the universe is compound interest." Based on the above calculations I would suggest that the fat-storing power of insulin is a close second. The good news is that we can prevent our fat cells from becoming sticky by making the right food choices.

4
Feed Your Brain...
or Suffer the Consequences

Sophie's Story

The day started like any other typical Monday as Sophie woke up and eyed her alarm clock as the dim early morning light filtered through her translucent drapes. She suddenly realized that she would be late for work yet again. While throwing on her clothes, hastily applying makeup and grabbing her briefcase on the way out the door, her mind was on a meeting she had to lead at the end of the day. She slipped into the old Toyota 4Runner that had been a gift from her dad when she graduated from college and deftly guided it toward the on ramp to I-70. The sun was low in the sky and she was heading directly into it.

At about that time she began feeling somewhat light-headed and woozy. Was this where she needed to turn? What a question for someone who had traveled the same route five days a week for the past 22 months. Oncoming cars appeared to be moving faster than she was used to. A vague, unsettling feeling was developing in the pit of her stomach, and it began to feel as if she were having an out-of-body experience. When a trickle of moisture appeared beneath her right armpit she realized that she was sweating, something she had never noticed before in the middle of winter.

In addition to that, a somewhat intangible nervousness had set in. This was a common occurrence when she had drunk too much coffee, but she didn't recall having had any this morning. The road appeared to be narrowing, and navigating between the closely spaced cars was becoming a chore. A simple trip to the office was beginning to feel like the Twilight Zone. Sophie's eyes were having trouble focusing, and her angst about being tardy for work took on a demeanor of unreality. An uneasiness settled upon her as the warmth of the electric car seat engulfed her.

The next thing she recalls was staring up into the eyes of a physician in the emergency room of the county hospital. It wasn't clear whether she was awake or if the whole thing was a dream. She was being asked to count backwards from ten, to squeeze the doctor's fingers and to follow a flashlight with her eyes. "Are you taking any medications? Do you have any allergies? What is your health like?" are the questions she heard being asked.

Not being fully coherent, it was unclear if *she* needed to respond or if the questions were directed at another person nearby. As her double vision cleared it became apparent she had an IV in and her vital signs were being monitored with electrical leads. At about that time a nurse came to her bedside and poked her finger with a needle to recheck her blood glucose level. As she was dozing back to sleep she was startled to hear, "54, you're headed in the right direction!"

Now feeling more alert, Sophie asked what had happened to her. "You have diabetes don't you?" the nurse asked.

"Well, yes," Sophie stammered in a concerned manner.

"It seems like you overdid it when you took your medicine today. When you arrived your blood sugar was about 30 and you weren't making much sense. Luckily we identified that and started an IV to give you some sugar water. It did the trick and you look much better now. By the way, the paramedics said when they arrived at the scene of the accident you had hit several cars and had come to rest in a large hedge. It was fortunate that nobody was injured."

In a startled fashion, Sophie responded, "Nothing like this has ever happened to me before. The funny part is that I don't remember a thing! I know I was in a hurry as I left for work and I must have taken too much insulin."

"You're going to be fine. But we'll have to watch you for a while to make sure your blood tests stabilize. However, we'll need to have a family member drive you home later in the day," said the nurse.

Too Much of a Good Thing

This scenario is played out with some regularity in many ERs throughout the country. One of the common side effects of an inadvertent overdose of insulin is hypoglycemia (low blood sugar). When an excessive amount of insulin is injected, it produces a large fall in blood glucose, or blood sugar as it is commonly called. What happened to Sophie is a typical result that illustrates an important lesson. The biological effect of insulin is to clear glucose (the main fuel for the brain) from the blood by transporting it into the muscles of the body. This is how insulin regulates blood sugar levels. However, as insulin transports glucose into muscle cells, it diverts it *away from the brain*. Since the brain depends on a continuous supply of glucose from the blood, in the presence of too much insulin the brain can suffer.

In people who don't have diabetes, blood glucose levels fluctuate throughout the day in relation to the types and amounts of food that are consumed. Diets that contain more sugar and foods that are rapidly broken down into glucose cause blood

As insulin transports glucose into muscle cells, it diverts it away from the brain.

glucose levels to rise. When this happens, the body's response is to release insulin. The greater the rise in blood glucose, the larger the stimulus is to release insulin. As insulin levels rise in the blood, glucose is transported out of the bloodstream into muscle cells. That is how the system works to control blood sugar.

Problems arise when "spikes" or dramatic rises in insulin levels occur. They can produce subsequent periods of hypoglycemia (low blood sugar) because the insulin stays in the bloodstream longer than glucose and it subsequently tends to drive glucose levels *below normal*. (Look at Figure 3.2 in Chapter 3 and see that Jane's glucose level went below normal at about 10:30) If these swings are mild you might only feel hungry. When they are more severe, it is not uncommon to feel shaky or jittery or to develop brain fog and not think clearly. When insulin levels are persistently elevated, or in people with blood sugar regulating problems, brain problems can be even more severe.

As you can see, what we eat determines how much insulin is released. In diabetics like Sophie who can't make any insulin because she developed juvenile diabetes, several daily insulin injections are required. They need to guess how much glucose-rich (meaning carbohydrate-containing) food will be consumed at a given meal and then calculate how much insulin to inject to "cover" the expected rise in blood sugar the meal will produce.

If insufficient insulin is administered, blood glucose levels remain elevated. If too much is given, glucose levels fall, sometimes so low that they cause tremulousness, jitteriness or difficulty thinking. If blood glucose levels fall further, coma may ensue.

This is exactly what happened to Sophie's brain. With too much insulin floating around, the glucose molecules were shunted away from her brain and into muscle cells. Under these circumstances, her brain didn't have sufficient glucose to convert to the energy it needed to keep functioning properly. This literally starved the brain cells and caused her to lose consciousness.

Since brain cells (or neurons as they are called) can't store glucose, they rely on a continuous supply from the blood. Sophie blacked out because of the hypoglycemia (low blood sugar) the insulin overdose caused. When that happens, it produces the equivalent of a brownout or energy failure and the brain can't operate normally. The less glucose that is available to the brain, the greater the brain starvation. This is exactly what happened to Sophie's neurons with catastrophic results.

Less dramatic swings in blood sugar can occur in people who don't have diabetes. They usually are caused by sugar binges followed shortly thereafter by a large insulin spike that produces effects similar to those Sophie experienced, although not as severe. However, as is evident, too much insulin—whether injected or in conjunction with poor dietary choices—can contribute to brain starvation.

Effect on the Brain

As Sophie learned, when insulin levels are high glucose (the main fuel of the brain) is directed *away from the brain* and into other tissues such as muscle. As we have seen previously, persistently elevated insulin also keeps fat locked in fat cells. This combination makes us fat *and* starves our brains by diverting nutrients away from neurons and into other cells for storage. Sophie's brain suffered the consequences. While swings in insulin might not be as dramatic in non-diabetic individuals, they occur nonetheless and can make us hungry and contribute to brain aging.

Too much insulin can contribute to brain starvation.

This is easily demonstrated by looking at statistics relating disorders of glucose and insulin metabolism to the incidence of the major neurodegenerative disorder being seen throughout the world—Alzheimer's disease (AD). Diabetics have four times the risk for developing AD; those with prediabetes have triple the risk and persons with pre-prediabetes (meaning that their blood sugar is normal all the time, but they have to work harder to control it by releasing more insulin throughout the day) have double the risk. These observations are a few of the reasons why many brain scientists around the world are beginning to refer to Alzheimer's disease as Type 3 diabetes. In Type 1 and Type 2 diabetes there is an inability to efficiently use glucose throughout the body. Type 3 diabetes refers to the same problem in the brain—with the consequences we have just discussed.

How to Prevent Alzheimer's Disease

Over the past ten years neuroscientists have identified an inability of the brain in Alzheimer's patients to properly use glucose. This has been documented by sensitive brain scans called PET (positron emission tomography) scans. In certain instances these changes can be seen decades before a diagnosis of Alzheimer's disease is made—suggesting to experts in this field that the inability of the brain to properly use glucose might be a key factor *in the development of the disease.*

To prevent diabetes of the brain and the body, it makes sense to select foods that feed the brain while maintaining stable blood sugar and insulin levels.

Part 2
Brain and Belly Friendly Diets

5

Feeding Your Brain *and* Losing Your Belly

I f it were true that eating too much is the only thing that makes you get fat, then consciously restricting food intake might make sense. But as we've seen by investigating John and Jane, the real problem is *sticky fat cells*. So making food choices that avoid them is the best way to stay thin and prevent calories from bypassing hungry brain cells—not forcing ourselves to eat less.

To see why, consider the following. What would happen if you continued to make poor food choices and, in addition, ate fewer calories? You would just get really hungry. Why? For two reasons. You're both eating less and storing many of the calories in a way that prevents you from using them. Let's look at an example.

Suppose that you need to *burn* 2,000 calories each day to meet the needs of your body and brain. If you choose foods that make your fat cells sticky, you'll store a number of those calories (say 200 for this discussion) in fat and won't be able to use them. That leaves 1,800 calories, which don't cover your metabolic requirements. If you also cut the number of calories you eat—say by 600 —you now, in effect, only have 1,200 (1,800 – 600) to get through the day. So all this approach will do is make you really hungry. How long do you think you'll stay on any diet that provides little more than 50 percent of the calories your body needs?

Now consider an alternative approach. Choose foods that prevent sticky fat cells from developing. *But don't cut calories!* Don't force yourself to eat less. What happens? First of all, you won't get hungry because you will be able to satisfy your metabolic requirements since you have access to all 2,000 of the calories you have eaten (because they are not locked away in your fat cells).

In addition, fat cells that aren't sticky actually release *additional* fat for your body to use. Suppose it amounts to about 300 fat calories a day. That plus the 2,000 calories you have eaten are now *more* than your body needs. As a result, your brain will sense these extra calories and will respond by *spontaneously decreasing your appetite* so you'll end up eating less. Why? Because you will be using internal calories from your "pantries" meaning you are burning your own fat. Thus, you will only need to eat 1,700 calories (2,000 – 300).

This is exactly what you need to do to lose weight—naturally, by reversing the hormonal abnormality that your previous food choices caused! Since high insulin levels are a major contributor to most increasing waistlines, this is the approach that makes the most sense.

To achieve the desired result you need to eat more fat (actually to include more of the *right* fats in your diet)—something that will dramatically curb appetite—and select foods that act as slow-release carb sources. When you do this, you'll avoid the sticky fat cell problem and you'll lose weight *without being constantly hungry or feeling like you're depriving yourself.*

Eat Fat to Lose Fat?

At this point you may be thinking, "It's all so confusing. If I want to get rid of fat, why is eating additional fat going to make me thinner? Won't I have to burn the fat that I eat *plus* what I'm already carrying around?"

The answer to that question is "yes." But to see why eating fat to lose fat makes sense, you must understand how fat is handled and how the hormonal changes that are induced actually produce weight loss. As we have already discussed, fat in the diet has essentially no effect on the level of insulin floating around in the blood. So eating more fat (while consuming the same number of calories) keeps insulin levels low and avoids the sticky fat cell problem.

Hence, if we eat *more of the right kind of fat* we eat less of the foods that cause insulin to increase. That is important for maintaining non-stick fat cells and controlling appetite. The other important goal is to carefully select what type of carbohydrates you eat. By including those that contain fiber (which slows their absorption—and as a result produces less impact on insulin), fat cells will be able to release fat to be burned.

Why does this approach speed up weight loss? It does so because it allows us to rely more on calories from our "pantries" and less on the foods we eat. Basically, we start to burn internal (stored) rather than external (eaten) calories. As we make this transition (which must happen if weight is to be lost), we spontaneously eat less because a larger proportion of the calories being burned come from our fat stores.

To put things another way, eating like this facilitates the metabolic transition that enables us to burn more stored fat by diminishing appetite (as demonstrated in the dietary analysis presented in Chapter 2). As hunger decreases the body naturally relies more on internal energy than on what we eat, which results in weight loss. When this happens without increasing appetite, *diets are easy to follow long term.*

Eat more of the right fats and select foods that act as slow-release carb sources. This will dramatically curb your appetite.

Is There Such a Thing as *Healthy Fat*?

If we ate no fat in our diet, we would develop what is referred to as a dietary deficiency disease. For example, a diet that contains no thiamin (a B vitamin) leads to the development of a disorder called beriberi (vitamin B1 deficiency) because B vitamins are *essential* nutrients in our diet—meaning that since our body can't make them, we must consume them each day or suffer the consequences.

There is an array of nutrients for which this is the case. They include vitamins (both fat and water soluble), certain amino acids (protein building blocks), minerals (such as calcium and magnesium) and certain other micronutrients including manganese, iron, selenium and chromium as well as many others.

Just as there are essential amino acids that our body can't make, there are also *essential fats* that fall into the same category. Hence, they *must* be included in the diet. Otherwise a deficiency disease will develop. For this reason they are referred to as essential fats and include linoleic acid (an omega-6 type of fat—one category of essential fat), α-linolenic acid (an omega-3 type of fat—the other category of essential fat) and their long-chain cousins arachidonic acid (an omega-6 fat found in meat, for example) and the omega-3 fat docosahexaenoic acid (DHA) found in cold-water fish. If these essential fats are not included in our diets, we will get sick.

As a matter of fact the omega-3 fats are so important that many experts in the field of child development believe that omega-3 fatty acid deficiency is a contributor to the epidemic of ADD/ADHD we are currently experiencing. Thus, fat is not only essential, it is necessary for the proper functioning of our most important organs.

In addition to the essential fats, many other types of fats play vital roles throughout our bodies. These are called *functional* fats because of the important metabolic roles they fulfill and *structural* fats due to the key role they play in the makeup of our cells and organelles (special compartments within cells).

Other types of fats are stored in our "pantries" as buffers against food shortages. There are even special types of fats that are preferentially burned rather than being stored and thus keep our energy levels up—clearly something that we should all be interested in. You have probably not heard much about this last category of special fats, but you will shortly.

Why Limit Fat?

If fat is so important, why have we been told for years to limit the amount of fat we eat? Good question! One possible answer is that if we want to lose fat, then we should eat less of it. The problem with this approach, as we have seen, is the adverse hormonal impact of doing so. In addition, we have all witnessed the disastrous health consequences of eating a low fat diet and know we must move on.

Each day fascinating nutritional information becomes available that allows us to make better decisions about what to eat. For example, many of the older nutritional recommendations didn't factor in the potent, inflammatory responses generated by the foods that were being recommended at the time. We are now aware of the central role that inflammation plays in heart disease, joint and bone degeneration and brain disorders.

During the last forty years—while the low-fat eating experiment was being conducted—obesity and diabetes rates soared. This suggests, among other things, that eating what constitutes a low-fat diet can be associated with excessive weight gain and all the diseases linked to it. It is time to revamp our thinking about fat, and in the context of the brain-belly connection it is most appropriate to do so. After all, the brain is mostly comprised of fat, which must be continuously replaced for optimal function.

If we need to eat more fat, what types and how much should be included?

Different Types of Fat

For the past four decades you might have thought there was a curse on fats, oils and oily foods. We have gone through various dietary phases during which recommendations have included restricted-fat diets, low-fat diets and very low-fat diets. Over this same period of time, belt and dress sizes have soared and obesity has become the norm rather than the exception.

However, just as all carbohydrates are not created equal, the same applies for fats. One type should be avoided at all costs. It is a category called *trans fats* and is listed collectively under the name *partially hydrogenated oils.* On food labels they typically appear as partially hydrogenated corn oil, partially hydrogenated sunflower oil or partially hydrogenated safflower oil. Food manufacturers use these manmade fats to extend the shelf life of packaged goods. The only problem is that they are unhealthy and can elevate LDL cholesterol (the "bad" cholesterol) and lower HDL cholesterol (the "good" cholesterol).

Not only are they bad for heart health, they are also bad for the brain because they counteract the beneficial actions of the healthy omega-3 fats. For these reasons trans fats should be on your list of foods to avoid completely. However, you need to read labels carefully to see where they are lurking. They are in everything from french fries to cookies.

The other type of fat that should be minimized, but not demonized, is animal fat that occurs in the form of the white, lard-like portion of roasts. It is basically a collection of (primarily) long-chain saturated fat molecules—a form of empty calorie storage—that is similar to what we store in our "pantries." It can easily be trimmed although leaving a bit of it adds to the flavor of the meat when it is cooked.

While intrinsically not too bad, it is a source of calories without much nutritional benefit—so why eat a lot of it in the first place? Having noted that, I'd like to mention several of its beneficial attributes including its ability to elevate HDL cholesterol (the "good" cholesterol). It is also one of the few ways to lower *lipoprotein a*—a potent risk factor for heart disease—something that no medications currently on the market can accomplish.

The Importance of "Balance"

The two types of essential fats—omega-3 and omega-6—are available in many foods. The problem is that they should be balanced in our diet, which means that they must be consumed in roughly equal amounts to keep their ratio close to 1:1. What has happened, largely due to the prevalence of vegetable oils on grocery store shelves, is that we eat far too much omega-6 oil and not enough omega-3. The impact of this dietary imbalance has produced omega-6/omega-3 ratios in the 20:1 range, which induces unhealthy inflammatory changes in our bodies. To normalize the ratio of essential fats we must markedly diminish omega-6 intake (see Table 5.1) and enhance omega-3 consumption (see Tables 5.2, 5.3, 5.4, 5.5 and 5.6).

Table 5.1: Omega-6 Fat Sources

Safflower oil	Sunflower oil	Corn oil	Soybean oil

Table 5.2: Omega-3 Fat Sources

Salmon	Bluefish	Walnuts
Herring	Tuna	Leafy greens
Sardines	Mackerel	Hemp seed oil
Halibut	Wild game such as venison and buffalo	Purslane
Anchovies	Flaxseeds and flaxseed oil	

Table 5.3: Content of Long-Chain Omega-3 Fat (grams) per 100-gram serving (about 3.5 ounces)

Atlantic Salmon (farmed)	1.8	Halibut	0.4
Anchovy (canned in oil)	1.7	Haddock	0.2
Sardine	1.4	Cod	0.1
Herring (pickled)	1.2	Mussel (blue)	0.7
Mackerel	1.0	Oyster	0.5
Trout (Rainbow, farmed)	1.0	Scallop	0.3
Swordfish	0.7	Clam	0.2
Tuna (white, canned in water)	0.7	Shrimp	0.3
Pollock	0.5		

(Source: USDA Nutrient Database for Standard Reference)

Table 5.4: Content of Shorter-Chain Omega-3 Fat (grams) per 1 ounce serving: Nuts and seeds

Almonds (dry roasted)	0.0	Pistachios (roasted)	0.1
Walnuts	2.6	Poppy seeds	0.1
Flax seeds	1.8	Pumpkin seeds (shelled)	0.1
Pecans (dry roasted)	0.3	Sesame seeds	0.1

(Source: Minnesota Nutrient Database 4.04 (last revised 3/02)

Table 5.5: Content of Shorter-Chain Omega-3 Fat (grams) per 1-tablespoon serving

Walnut oil	1.4	Canola oil	1.3
Soybean oil (unhydrogenated)	0.9	Olive oil	0.1
Flax seed oil	6.9		

(Source: Minnesota Nutrient Database 4.04 (last revised 3/02)

Table 5.6: Content of Shorter-Chain Omega-3 Fat (grams) per 1-cup serving

Spinach (fresh, cooked)	0.2	Kale (cooked)	0.2
Green leaf lettuce	trace	Collard greens (cooked)	0.2
Dandelion greens (cooked)	0.2		

(Source: Minnesota Nutrient Database 4.04 (last revised 3/02)

MUFAs

Monounsaturated fat (see Table 5.7) is a very healthy type of fat. It is a liquid at room temperature and becomes thicker or even semi-solid when refrigerated. Olive oil is a common example of oil that contains monounsaturated fatty acids (MUFAs). MUFAs help lower "bad" cholesterol without affecting levels of "good" cholesterol.

They can even speed up belly fat loss. In one study, dieters who consumed MUFAs lost *56 percent more central body fat than those on a low fat diet.* And this was accomplished *without cutting calories or doing additional exercise!* Findings in another study showed that a meal containing MUFAs enhanced fat burning for the next five hours.

MUFAs also help normalize blood sugar levels—in a very unusual manner. When intake of MUFAs is increased, the body produces more of a hormone called *adiponectin.* Higher levels of it are beneficial because adiponectin improves glucose metabolism.

Table 5.7: Good MUFA Sources

Oils (1 Tbsp contains 120 calories)	Nuts (½ oz)	Other
Olive oil	Almonds, 82 calories	1 olive, 10 calories
Flax oil	Brazil nuts, 85 calories	¼ medium avocado,
Sesame oil	Hazelnuts, 79 calories	70 calories
Walnut oil	Cashews dry roasted, 82 calories	½ oz dark chocolate
	Macadamias, dry roasted, 101 calories	143 calories
	Walnuts, 92 calories	
	Pistachios, dry roasted, 80 calories	

Coconut—The Miracle Oil!

The numerous benefits of coconut oil are finally being recognized. They include its unique ability to promote a healthy metabolism and provide almost immediate energy. In addition, it is the best cooking oil on the planet! Olive oil is good, but coconut oil is truly superb. Its delicate taste will enhance anything you are cooking and it is not damaged by heat.

You might hear people say that coconut oil contains the most saturated fat of any edible oil. However, not all saturated fats are created equal. They come in different lengths. Long-chain saturated fats are primarily stored in the body in fat tissue.

However, most of the fats in coconut oil are *medium-chain* lengths and are called medium-chain triglycerides (MCTs). When they are eaten, they go directly to the liver where they are converted into a readily available energy source rather than being stored as fat. In fact, the MCTs in coconut oil can *actually stimulate your metabolism, leading to weight loss!*

This was discovered serendipitously back in the 1940s when farmers tried to use inexpensive coconut oil to fatten their livestock. To their surprise, what they discovered was that the cattle became leaner, not fatter. Since then, numerous studies have shown that you lose weight when you replace long-chain fat (saturated or unsaturated) in your diet with the same amount of medium-chain fat.

The MCTs in coconut oil are metabolized into compounds called *ketone bodies*, also known as *ketones*. We will see how ketones are brain savers and can be used easily by neurons to decrease appetite and sharpen focus, memory and concentration.

The bottom line is to add coconut oil to your diet for a host of reasons.

A Match Made in Heaven

Usually only DHA (docosahexaenoic acid) is mentioned when one discusses omega-3 fatty acids and the brain. This is because it keeps the membranes of our nerve cells soft and flexible, traits that allow them to be exquisitely responsive to the trillions of signals they must process. Make no mistake; DHA is vital for a healthy brain. However, based on recent findings from Dr. Stephen

Cunnane, a noted Canadian expert on diet and nutrition, other omega-3 fats are just as important for the brain.

DHA's shorter relative—α-linolenic acid—must now be visualized from an entirely new perspective. In addition to being a precursor for DHA (meaning it can be chemically transformed into DHA by the body), Dr. Cunnane's novel observations have demonstrated that it can also be metabolized into ketones. Ketones are a unique fuel for the brain. Why? Because it can turn them into energy as efficiently as glucose.

This means ketones can be used as brain food in addition to, or instead of, glucose. So, whenever glucose is in short supply, ketones can fill in—and as a ready source of ketones, α-linolenic acid can supply this much-needed energy. Sources of α-linolenic acid (the shorter-chain omega-3 fat) are listed in Tables 5.4, 5.5 and 5.6.

An example of how this interaction works might be helpful. As was demonstrated when Sophie took too much insulin, if the brain is exposed to a glucose shortage it immediately malfunctions because of the lack of energy. However, if ketones are present they can be used as an alternative source of energy by nerve cells even when glucose isn't available.

Since the brain doesn't care where the energy comes from (glucose or ketones), when glucose isn't available, ketones can easily fill in. When this happens, there is no power shortage and no symptoms develop. Under these circumstances, the brain functions fine without any interruption. Thus, ketones can prevent brain starvation. This has several beneficial implications. When neurons are properly fed, two good things happen—we don't get hungry and we think more clearly!

Ketones can be used easily by neurons to decrease appetite and sharpen focus, memory and concentration.

To underscore how effective this approach is, let's consider a new product on the market that is a medical food called Axona™. A *medical food* is prescribed by a doctor for the treatment of a medical condition. In this instance, Axona™ is used for the treatment of moderate to severe Alzheimer's disease. It can be used with any of the other Alzheimer drugs on the market because it works in a different manner. It allows the brain cells to generate more energy and hence function better. It performs this miraculous feat by producing large amounts of brain-friendly ketones.

Ketones and the Brain–Belly Connection

It is the energy the ketones generate that is important. The brain can't tell whether its energy is coming from glucose or ketones…and it doesn't really care. All that matters is that it is provided with all the energy it needs. As long as there is gas in the tank, so to speak, the brain considers itself well fed. Under these circumstances there is no brain starvation and we don't get hungry! So, as a consequence, we don't overeat!

Other Sources

In addition to including coconut oil and the universe of omega-3 foods containing α-linolenic acid in your diet, there are other simple ways to increase the ability of your body to generate ketones internally. Not surprisingly, they are part of the Feed Your Brain Lose Your Belly diet program. Since ketones are generated when fat is being burned in the liver (an organ in the right upper part of the abdominal cavity), anything that facilitates fat burning will generate more ketones.

Ketones are naturally present in abundance during periods of starvation. This is a time when we rely almost exclusively on fat from our "pantries." During prolonged food shortages, insulin levels fall for this very reason. So, eating to minimize insulin, in addition to all of its other health benefits, naturally stimulates ketone formation. It involves choosing the right carbohydrates—

those that are slowly digested and produce minimal blood sugar fluctuations—usually the ones with higher fiber content. We will get into the "nuts and bolts" of which they are shortly.

Making the Best Food Choices

The Feed Your Brain Lose Your Belly diet doesn't require you to weigh, measure or count what you eat. It relies on making food choices that prevent the development of sticky fat cells. This, in turn, has a potent appetite suppressant effect. So you will naturally eat less because you are burning more stored calories.

By making the right food choices, how much you eat usually takes care of itself. As you enjoy meals containing high quality lean protein and healthy fats along with nutrient and fiber rich foods, you'll have little desire to overeat. On this program you'll get in touch with your body and be able to distinguish feeling hungry from wanting to eat, emotional eating, eating because you're depressed or bored or eating just for the sake of eating. Once you become attuned to the sometimes subtle signals you will be receiving, you'll only eat what you need. However, it doesn't mean that calories don't count. For this reason, I have made *suggestions* about portion sizes to be used as guidelines for the more calorie dense foods in the fat and oil categories.

As a rough guide, I recommend that about 20 percent of daily calories come from protein and that fat calories contribute 45 to 55 percent. This means that carbohydrates comprise about 25 to 35 percent of daily calorie content. Remember that these are guidelines, not rigid mandates. We're all different and amounts and quantities can vary from day to day. What are more important are the *food choices* you make, not the exact proportions.

To get started, I suggest that you include lean protein, slow-release carb choices and herbs and spices with each meal. Try to incorporate 5 servings (⅔ cup) of veggies from the Good Foods categories each day and a couple from the fruit (½ cup) category.

Eat good fats at each meal. Because of their calorie dense nature, I have provided guidelines about serving sizes for the fat/oil groups. Choose primarily from the mono-unsaturated fat group. Include sources of cold-water fish containing long-chain omega-3 fat several times a week. Add flaxseeds or flax oil every day. Get creative about the use of coconut oil.

For example, mix ½ tablespoon of flaxseed oil with 1½ tablespoons of olive oil and some balsamic vinegar, salt, pepper and fennel in salad dressing. Include three or four avocado slices with some rosemary chicken and asparagus with a drizzle of butter and fresh dill for lunch. Mix a tablespoon of coconut oil with some half-and-half in a bowl of steel cut oats sprinkled with cinnamon and topped with strawberries while enjoying a hard-boiled egg for breakfast. Savor a small handful of nuts (15), several small squares of cheese and a few grapes for an afternoon snack.

See the boxes that follow for the GOOD FOODS to choose from and the BAD FOODS to avoid. Be creative. Make selections you haven't tried before. Experiment with an array of colors, shapes and sizes. Strive to make the food look as good as it tastes. Choose fruits and veggies from many cultures! Don't forget the herbs and spices, which are virtually calorie free and contain an almost endless supply of valuable phytonutrients such as antioxidants (free-radical fighters) and anti-inflammatories. Spend time learning how to combine them in unexpected ways. Doing so can dramatically alter the taste of a dish that has become boring or not very stimulating. Mix spicy and sharp with sweet and mild. Use coconut oil for cooking and add it to other dishes for its delicate flavor.

To help facilitate better carb choices, a discussion of the glycemic index (GI) concept will be helpful. The glycemic index is a number assigned to foods that contain carbohydrates—the triggers that raise glucose and insulin levels—that helps guide food choices by providing a relative rating scale that reflects the impact of each food on blood sugar. (Note that fat and protein don't impact blood sugar and are not on the GI list.)

GOOD FOODS

VEGETABLES

(good slow-release carbohydrates)

Artichoke hearts	Jicama
Arugula	Kale
Asparagus	Kohlrabi
Bok choi	Leeks
Broccoli	Lettuce
Brussels sprouts	Mushrooms
Cabbage	Okra
Cauliflower	Onions
Celery	Peppers
Chard	Radishes
Collard greens	Scallions
Cucumbers	Shallots
Eggplant	Spinach
Endive	Squash
Green and yellow	Tomatoes
beans	Turnip greens
Hearts of palm	Watercress

LEGUMES

Black beans	Italian beans
Black-eyed peas	Kidney beans
Broad beans	Lentils
Butter beans	Lima beans
Chickpeas	Navy beans
(garbanzos)	Pinto beans
Edamame	Soybeans

FRUIT

(Note: fruit can be high in sugar content so I suggest 2 servings per day with sizes as shown below)

Apple, 1
Apricots, 4 fresh or 6 dried
Banana, ½
Blackberries, ½ cup
Blueberries, ½ cup
Cantaloupe, 1 small slice
Cherries, 15
Clementine, 1
Cranberries, ½ cup
Grapefruit, ¼
Grapes, 10
Honeydew, 1 small slice
Kiwi, ½
Mango, ⅙
Nectarine, ½
Orange, 1
Peach, ½
Pear, ¼
Plum, 1
Prune, 2
Raspberries, ½ cup
Strawberries, ½ cup
Tangerine, 1

It is determined by feeding humans who have fasted overnight a 50-gram portion of the desired food. Blood samples are then drawn every 15 minutes for three hours. These values are then plotted on a graph. The resultant curve reflects the impact of that food on subsequent blood sugar level. It is then compared with the graph obtained after a 50-gram glucose meal, which is rated arbitrarily as being 100. Generally speaking, the lower the GI rating the lower the impact of the food on blood glucose levels.

Numbers over 70 are high, those under 55 are good and those below 30 are very good.

The GI of each food that contains carbohydrates has been calculated. For example, glucose is rated at 100. Corn flakes are 98. A French baguette is 95. A baked potato is 93. Whole wheat bread is 77. A donut is 76. Popcorn is 72. Pizza is 60. Raisins are 56. Strawberries are 42. Lentils are 30. Cherries are 22. Broccoli is 10. I have included a more complete listing of the GI of a number of foods on the next page.

Note: The glycemic index (GI) has been criticized for the following reasons:

◊ It does not take into account other health-related factors in the interpretation of the glycemic response to carbohydrates (such as the insulin response).

◊ The GI is significantly altered by the state of the food such as ripeness, processing, storage and cooking methods (such as baked potatoes vs. mashed potatoes vs. fried potatoes).

◊ The GI varies from person to person.

◊ Sugars such as fructose have a low GI, but when used excessively (more than 4 grams per day) are bad for your health for other reasons (such as contributing to the development of insulin resistance, diabetes and obesity). The take-home message is that sugars should be avoided even though some of them have a low GI.

Table 5.8: Glycemic Index (GI)

Ranges of GI: Very low GI (10–30) Low GI (35–55)
Medium GI (60–69) High GI (70 and above)

Cereals
Corn Flakes. 98
Rice Crispies 100
Muesli 68

Grains
Buckwheat 54
Bulgur 48
Brown rice 55
Short grain white rice . 72

Dairy
Milk (whole). 22
Milk (skimmed). . . . 32
Ice cream (whole). . 61
Ice cream (low fat) . 50
Yogurt (low fat). . . . 33

Cookies
Graham crackers . . . 74
Melba Toast. 70
Oatmeal cookies. . . 55
Rice cakes 82
Rice crackers 91
Soda crackers. 74
Stoned wheat thins 67

Snack foods
Corn chips 72
Jelly beans 80
Popcorn 72
Pretzels 83
Chocolate bar 49

Breads
Bagel 72
Blueberry muffin. . . 59
Croissant. 67
Donut. 76
Pita bread. 57
Sour dough 52
Rye bread. 76
Stone ground
whole wheat 53
Pumpernickel. 51
White. 70

Fruit
Apple. 38
Banana. 55
Cantaloupe 65
Cherries. 22
Grapefruit. 25
Grapes. 46
Kiwi 52
Mango. 55
Orange 44
Papaya. 58
Pear 38
Pineapple 66
Plum. 39
Raisins 56
Strawberries. 42
Watermelon. 103

Vegetables
Beets 69
Broccoli. 10
Cabbage. 10
Carrots. 49
Corn. 55
Green peas. 48
Lettuce 10
Mushrooms 10
Onions. 10
Parsnips. 97
Potato (baked) 93
Potato (instant,
mashed) 86
Potato (new) 62
Potato (French fries)75
Red peppers 10
Pumpkin 75
Sweet potato. 54

Pasta
Spaghetti. 43
Fettuccini. 32
Spiral pasta. 43
Capellini 45
Linguini 46
Macaroni. 47
Rice vermicelli. 58

Beans
Baked beans. 48
Broad beans. 79
Garbanzo beans
(chickpeas). 33
Lentils 30
Lima beans 32
Navy beans 38
Pinto beans 39
Red kidney beans. . 27
Soy beans. 18
White beans 31

Sugars
Fructose 23
Glucose 100
Honey 58
Lactose 46
Maltose 105
Sucrose
(table sugar). 65

Table 5.9: Nuts, Seeds, Oils and Other Fats
(Remember that these are calorie dense foods. Numbers are suggested serving sizes. Two to three servings of nuts or seeds are recommended per day.)

Nuts and Seeds	Oils
Almonds. 15	MUFA containing oils
Brazil nuts. 4	Canola
Cashews 15	Olive
Filberts 20	Products containing polyunsaturated
Flaxseed . . . . 3 Tbsp	oils
Hazelnuts. 20	(Use sparingly)
Macadamia nuts. 9	Corn
Pecans. 12	Peanut
Pine nuts. . . . . .1 oz	Safflower
Pistachios 25	Sesame
Pumpkin seeds . . . . . 3 Tbsp	Soybean
Sesame seeds . . . . . . 3 Tbsp	Sunflower
Sunflower seeds. . . . 3 Tbsp	Specialty Oils (Try to include 1 or 2
Walnuts. 15	Tbsp per day of each)
	Flaxseed
	Coconut (an excellent cooking oil)

Other Fats
Avocado (¼ to ½ whole or 1 Tbsp oil)
Olives (5–10, or ½ Tbsp oil) (If in salad dressing, use 2 Tbsp)
Butter (1 or 2 pats per day)
Margarine (trans fat free, 1 or 2 pats per day)

Benefits of Herbs and Spices

These tasty seasonings can add much more than flavor, color and variety to your favorite foods. Every time you flavor your meals with herbs and spices you are literally making whatever you eat "better" without adding a single calorie. Here are some reasons why:

◊ They maximize nutrient density because they contain vitamins, minerals, and anti-oxidants.

◊ They make the diet more thermogenic (by increasing your metabolism), which means that you burn calories faster.

Table 5.10: Herbs and Spices (Use liberally, mix freely, and be creative!)

Allspice	Cinnamon	Oregano
Anise	Clove	Paprika
Basil	Coriander	Parsley
Bay leaf	Cumin	Pepper
Caraway	Dill	Poppy seed
Cardamom	Dill seed	Red pepper
Cayenne pepper	Fennel	Rosemary
Celery seed	Garlic	Saffron
Chervil	Ginger	Sage
Chicory	Horseradish	Thyme
Chili pepper	Mace	Turmeric
Chili powder	Marjoram	Vanilla
Chives	Mustard	Wasabi
Cilantro	Nutmeg	

◊ Some even make you feel fuller. One study demonstrated that eating ½ teaspoon of red pepper flakes before a meal decreased subsequent calorie intake by 10 to 15 percent.

◊ The complex flavors they impart decrease the need for salt.

◊ Certain spices (such as cinnamon and coriander) allow your body to handle glucose more effectively.

◊ Others (cumin, sage and turmeric) improve brain health.

◊ Basil, cinnamon, thyme, saffron and ginger have immune boosting powers.

Many have distinctive health-promoting properties as well. Here are some of my favorites and what they "bring to the table."

Ginger

The active ingredient in ginger is gingerol, a compound that is believed to relax blood vessels and relieve pain. One of its most well-known benefits is to ameliorate motion sickness, nausea and vomiting. For these reasons it is helpful to people suffering from the side effects of cancer chemotherapy.

It is also anti-inflammatory, which means it may be helpful in fending off heart disease and arthritis and is chock full of antioxidants that are powerful free radical fighters. Free radicals are damaging chemical compounds that are generated by our bodies each day. They can break down the delicate fats, proteins and genetic material in our cells.

Ginger can be used freshly ground from the root. It is also served with sushi. Fresh ginger root even makes a soothing ginger tea. Dried ground ginger is typically used in baking.

Cinnamon

People with diabetes should be particularly aware that cinnamon is a useful tool to help control blood sugar. A study reported in the 2004 issue of *Diabetes Care* found that this tasty spice acts to prevent the development of insulin resistance—a condition that contributes to the abnormal blood sugar swings so characteristic of diabetes. It also reduces total cholesterol levels, LDL cholesterol ("bad" cholesterol) and triglycerides.

A study in the *Journal of Nutrition* found that cinnamon is one of the best sources of disease fighting antioxidants.

It comes in sticks and as a powder. It can be used as a garnish, sprinkled atop a bowl of oatmeal, grated over espresso drinks and as a spice to help flavor curries and vegetables.

Turmeric

Curcumin is the component that gives turmeric its bright yellow color. It is a potent anti-inflammatory compound that is the likely source of turmeric's benefits in inflammatory bowel disorders, cancer and Alzheimer's disease.

Turmeric powder has a warm, peppery flavor similar to ginger and orange. It is used in curries, egg salad, bean dishes, salad dressings and sauces.

Sage

Sage also has antioxidant and anti-inflammatory properties. It seems to promote better brain function, as documented by a study in the June, 2003 issue of *Pharmacological Biochemical Behavior* that found significantly enhanced recall in subjects who received sage oil compared to those who received placebo product.

Its slightly sweet flavor makes it quite versatile. Sage can be added to soups, salad dressings and sauces or sprinkled over vegetables.

Parsley

Parsley is a rich source of antioxidants and other heart-protective nutrients including vitamin C and folic acid. Animal studies using parsley have shown that it can inhibit tumor formation and can neutralize carcinogens including those found in cigarette smoke.

Fresh parsley is much more flavorful than the dried variety. It is used in salads, soups and casseroles and as a topping on fish and meat dishes. Try it as a breath freshener at the end of a meal, too!

Oregano

Oregano contains thymol and carvacrol—potent antibacterial compounds. It, too, is a powerful antioxidant and is rich in phyto-nutrients (beneficial plant nutrients). On a per gram basis fresh oregano has:

◊ 42 times more antioxidant activity than apples

◊ 12 times more than oranges

◊ 4 times more than blueberries

Fresh or dried oregano can be added to Italian dishes, salad dressings, egg dishes, vegetables and much more!

Table 5.11: Meat, Seafood, Cheese and Dairy

Beef	Poultry
(All lean cuts)	Cornish hen
Chuck	Turkey
Chuck eye	Chicken
Top blade	Pheasant
Pot roast	**Other Meat**
Short ribs	Pork
Brisket	Ham
Rib	Canadian bacon
Rib roast	Pork loin
Rib eye	Pork tenderloin
Back ribs	Veal
Short loin	Lamb
T-Bone	Game meats
Porterhouse	Buffalo
Tenderloin	Elk
Plate	Ostrich
Short steak	Venison
Flank	Yak
Flank steak	Soy-based meat substitutes
Sirloin	
Top sirloin	**Cheese**
Sirloin	(Most are fine, but limit to
Tri-Tip	an ounce per day)
Rounds	
Round steak	**Dairy**
Top round roast	(Avoid any that contain trans fats,
Top round steak	or added sugar or HFCS)
Bottom round roast	Milk (skim, 1%, 2%, or
Boneless rump roast	whole)
Ground beef	Plain yogurt
Pastrami	Half-and-half

Table 5.12: Beverages

Water
Coffee (caffeinated or decaf)
Tea
Diet soda
Wine (1–2 glasses (4 oz. each) at dinner, if desired)

BAD FOODS
(Limit or avoid entirely)

Bread
Rolls
Cake
Candy
Cookies
Honey
Sugar
High fructose corn
    syrup (HFCS)

Soda
Pasta (OK in small
    amounts, al dente
    is better)
White or red
    potatoes
Rice
Corn
Ice cream

Jam and jelly
Dates
Figs
Watermelon
Any foods containing
    trans fats

TREATS

Chocolate (limit to 1 oz
dark chocolate)

ARTIFICIAL SWEETENERS

(Use sparingly)

Sucralose (Splenda)
Acesulfame K
Aspartame (NutraSweet, Equal)
Saccharin (Sweet 'N Low)

The primary tenet of the diet is to include healthy fats and slow-release types of carbohydrates in a caloric ratio of greater than 2 to 1.

THE 12 ESSENTIAL COMPONENTS OF THE
FEED YOUR BRAIN LOSE YOUR BELLY DIET PROGRAM

◊ The primary tenet of the diet is to include healthy fats and slow-release types of carbohydrates in a caloric ratio (fat to carb) of greater than 2 to 1.

◊ Fish is brain food. It is also a key food source for fat loss. Have fish several times per week. Choose fatty, cold-water species such as trout, salmon, tuna, mackerel, herring, sardines, anchovies and halibut.

◊ Add lean protein from both animal and plant sources. Eggs are a wonderful source of protein as well as long-chain omega-3 fatty acids. Some are even supplemented with extra DHA.

◊ Incorporate sources of the shorter-chain omega-3 fat α-linolenic acid, which occurs most abundantly in ground flax seeds or flax seed oil. It is also present in walnuts (or walnut oil), wheat germ, pumpkin seeds, spirulina, purslane, parsley, broccoli, kale, spinach, cabbage, dark green leafy vegetables and Brussels sprouts.

◊ Include veggies and some fruits in the diet. Choose non-starchy varieties and berries of all sorts.

◊ Nuts and seeds typically contain mono-unsaturated fats and are generally good sources of potassium and magnesium. They are calorie dense, so go lightly and choose from a variety including almonds, pistachios, walnuts, pecans and cashews. Sunflower, sesame and pumpkin are my favorite seeds. They may be eaten plain or included in salads and casseroles.

◊ Spice up your diet. Herbs and spices make almost anything taste better and are anti-oxidant powerhouses that are calorie free.

◊ Blend color into the diet by selecting fruits and veggies in all hues of the rainbow. Be sure to mix and match because different colors provide different nutrients.

◊ Add avocadoes. They are an excellent source of mono-unsaturated fat, protein, vitamins and minerals. Have a slice with salad; add as a side dish with the main entrée or as a snack with berries.

◊ Don't forget coconut oil, which is the best cooking oil and a great source of energy because of its high content of medium-chain triglycerides (which also act as a powerful appetite suppressant).

◊ Green tea is a super beverage—so, enjoy it. Drink it hot or cold!

◊ Have a glass of red wine, if you like!

6
Seven-Day Meal Plan and Recipes

I n this chapter you'll find a varied array of dishes that I have enjoyed over the years. As you read through the recipes, please remember two things: 1) that the brain, which is made of fat, requires a continuous supply of healthy fatty nutrients in the diet for optimal functioning, and 2) that over the past 30 to 40 years during the low-fat eating experiment, obesity and diabetes have become commonplace. If eating less fat has contributed to this disastrous situation, eating more of the right type of fat should certainly help, as we have discussed repeatedly throughout this book.

Day 1: 1933 calories (fat 1012, 52%; carb 466, 24%; protein 455, 24%)
Fat to carb ratio: 2.2:1

BREAKFAST 1	Frozen Berry Smoothie (1 serving)
Calories 453 Fat 113 cal Carb 182 cal Protein 158 cal	1 cup frozen berries (strawberries, blueberries or mixed berries) ½ banana 1 cup water ½ cup ice 1 cup regular cottage cheese ½ cup 2% milk 1 tablespoon ground flax seeds Place all ingredients in a blender. Blend until the mixture is smooth and creamy. Pour and enjoy. This is one of my favorites. You can use raspberries, blueberries, strawberries, blackberries or substitute/mix in other berries.

LUNCH 1
 	
Calories 515
  Fat   385 cal
  Carb   71 cal
  Protein   59 cal
	Nectarine Ginger Chicken Salad (4 servings)
	3 nectarines (about 2.5 inches in diameter), sliced
	2 skinless chicken breasts, cooked and thinly sliced
	1 cup thinly sliced celery
	1 cup thinly sliced almonds
	¼ cup thinly sliced scallions
	
	  Combine the ingredients in a salad bowl. Add the dressing and toss lightly. Serve immediately.
	
	Dressing
	1 cup mayonnaise
	2 tablespoons white wine vinegar
	1 tablespoon honey
	½ teaspoon curry powder
	½ teaspoon ground ginger
	¼ teaspoon salt
	
	  Combine ingredients and mix thoroughly.

SNACK 1
 	
Calories 339
  Fat   227 cal
  Carb   77 cal
  Protein   35 cal
	(1 serving)
	1 Gala apple
	1 cube sharp Cheddar cheese (1 inch on a side)
	¼ cup walnut halves

DINNER 1
 	
Calories 696
  Fat   287 cal
  Carb   148 cal
  Protein 191 cal
	Broiled Minty Tuna (1 serving)
	1 tuna steak (1 inch thick; about 6 ounces)
	½ tablespoon olive oil
	⅛ teaspoon salt
	¼ clove garlic, minced
	¼ tablespoon soy sauce
	4 leaves fresh mint, chopped
	rosemary to taste
	lemon wedges
	
	  About 30 to 45 minutes before cooking, rub the tuna lightly with the olive oil and salt and let stand. Mix the garlic, soy sauce, mint, and rosemary. Immediately prior to cooking, rub the seasonings into the tuna. Broil 2 minutes per side. Serve with lemon wedges.

Include veggies and some fruits in the diet.
Choose nonstarchy varieties and berries of all sorts.

DINNER 1, Cont.	**Broiled Asparagus Stalks (1 serving)**

Broiled Asparagus Stalks (1 serving)
6 stalks fresh asparagus
1 teaspoon olive oil
1 teaspoon balsamic vinegar
salt and pepper to taste
cayenne pepper

Place the asparagus stalks on a baking sheet. Coat with a mixture of the olive oil and balsamic vinegar. Add salt and pepper and sprinkle very lightly with cayenne pepper. Broil for about 4 minutes.

Sautéed Yellow Squash with Gruyère Cheese (4 servings)
4 small yellow squash, thinly sliced
¼ cup butter
½ fresh sweet onion, thinly sliced
1 clove garlic, minced
2 tablespoons chopped fresh tarragon
¼ cup chopped fresh basil
2 ounces Gruyère cheese, thinly sliced
salt and pepper to taste

Melt the butter in a large sauté pan on fairly high heat. Coat the bottom of the pan evenly. Add the sliced squash and onions. Spread them out and cook them evenly, stirring frequently until very lightly browned at least on one side (about 2 minutes). Sprinkle with salt and pepper while cooking. About halfway through, add the garlic and herbs. Remove the pan from the heat and place the slices of cheese over the squash in a single layer. Let sit for a few minutes until just melted. Serve immediately.

Dessert: Cantaloupe with Cardamom (1 serving)
1 cup chilled cantaloupe balls
¼ teaspoon ground cardamom
½ teaspoon fresh lime juice
4 to 5 chocolate shavings

Mix the melon balls, lime juice, and cardamom. Serve in a glass dish with a mint leaf and chocolate.

Day 2: 1918 calories (fat 1021, 57%; carb 573, 29%; protein 324, 17%)
Fat to carb ratio: 1.8:1

BREAKFAST 2 Calories 489 Fat 274 cal Carb 171 cal Protein 44 cal	**Yogurt with Fruit and Nuts (1 serving)** 1 cup plain yogurt ¼ cup raisins ½ ounce sliced pecans 1 tablespoon flaxseed oil almond flavoring—drizzle to taste ground cinnamon to taste Mix yogurt, raisins, pecans, and flaxseed oil together in a bowl. Drizzle with almond flavoring, sprinkle with cinnamon and enjoy! This is a great breakfast that is well suited for the on-the-go lifestyle.

LUNCH 2
 	
Calories 476
Fat   253 cal
Carb   130 cal
Protein 93 cal
	Smoked Turkey Tortilla Wrap (1 serving)
	1 whole wheat tortilla
	3 slices of smoked turkey breast
	3 slices of avocado
	1 tablespoon sour cream
	¼ cup shredded Swiss cheese
	¼ cup salsa
	oregano
	
	   Heat tortilla in a skillet over medium heat until lightly browned. Arrange turkey strips, avocado slices, sour cream cheese and salsa over tortilla. Sprinkle lightly with oregano.
	   Roll and serve.

SNACK 2 Calories 345 Fat 154 cal Carb 161 cal Protein 30 cal	**Trail Mix (1 serving)** pumpkin seeds lightly toasted and salted (about 20 seeds) ¼ Cup dried sweetened cranberries ¼ Cup toasted shelled pistachios 10 Dark chocolate bits Mix together and enjoy!

DINNER 2	

DINNER 2

Calories 608
  Fat   340 cal
  Carb   111 cal
  Protein 157 cal

Lamb Chop with Herbs (1 serving)
1 lamb chop
2 pats butter, melted
chopped fresh rosemary
dill seed
garlic powder
sage
mint

  Mix the butter, rosemary, dill seed, garlic, sage and mint and brush on the lamb chop. Broil or grill to taste.

Sautéed Peppers (1 serving)
½ cup chopped red and yellow bell peppers
1 teaspoon hazelnut oil
1 teaspoon chopped fresh fennel

  Mix the peppers in a skillet, cover with the hazlenut oil and sauté. Sprinkle with fennel and serve immediately.

Spinach (1 serving)
1½ cups spinach
1 tablespoon olive oil
1 teaspoon lightly toasted sesame seeds

  Sauté the spinach very lightly in the oil. Top with the sesame seeds.

Dessert: Broiled pineapple (1 serving)
1 wedge fresh pineapple
cinnamon to taste

  Sprinkle pineapple with cinnamon and broil until lightly brown

Add lean protein from both animal and plant sources. Eggs are a wonderful source of protein as well as long-chain omega-3 fatty acids. Some are even supplemented with extra DHA.

Day 3: 1793 calories (fat 997, 55%; carb 427, 24%; protein 369, 21%)
Fat to carb ratio: 2.3:1

BREAKFAST 3	Southwestern Ham and Cheese Omelet (1 serving)
Calories 556 Fat 265 cal Carb 131 cal Protein 160 cal	2 eggs ¼ cup 2% milk butter for sautéing 2 ounces ham or Canadian bacon (sliced) 1 ounce grated Cheddar cheese 1 tablespoon salsa 1 slice sourdough toast with butter Whip the eggs. Add the milk. While cooking them in the butter, add Canadian bacon and cheese. Top with salsa. Serve with buttered sourdough toast.
LUNCH 3	Healthy Spinach Salad (1 serving)
Calories 459 Fat 268 cal Carb 100 cal Protein 91 cal	1½ cups spinach 1 carrot, grated 1 tomato, sliced 1 mushroom, sliced 4 ounces diced turkey sunflower seeds (about 10) raspberries (5) ⅛ cup sliced walnuts salt and pepper to taste Toss together the spinach, carrot, tomato, mushroom and turkey. Top with dressing (see below) and sprinkle with sunflower seeds, raspberries, walnuts, salt and pepper. **Salad Dressing (1 serving)** 1 tablespoon olive oil 1 teaspoon white wine vinegar ¼ teaspoon freshly squeezed lemon juice salt, pepper, celery seed and paprika to taste Mix the ingredients and shake well. Pour over the salad and serve immediately.
SNACK 3	Crackers and Nut Butter (1 serving)
Calories 223 Fat 157 cal Carb 31 cal Protein 35 cal	4–5 Blue Diamond Nut Thin crackers peanut or almond butter Spread crackers thinly with nut butter.

DINNER 3

Calories 555
- Fat   307 cal
- Carb   165 cal
- Protein   83 cal

Garlic Shrimp with Parsley (6 servings)

1½ pounds of medium shrimp, peeled and deveined
⅓ cup butter
4 medium cloves garlic, crushed and minced
⅓ cup fresh chopped parsley
2½ tablespoons freshly squeezed lemon juice
salt to taste

In a large skillet heat the butter over medium heat until it stops foaming (30 to 45 seconds). Add the shrimp and garlic and sauté, turning frequently until shrimp just turn pink (4 to 5 minutes). Add the parsley, lemon juice and salt and stir well. Remove the pan from the heat and serve.

Brussels Sprouts with Hazelnuts (6 servings)

1 tablespoon butter
1 pound Brussels sprouts, trimmed and quartered
¼ cup chopped hazelnuts
¼ teaspoon salt
freshly ground pepper to taste
3 tablespoons water

Preheat the oven to 450°F. Position the rack in the lower third of oven. Place the butter on a rimmed baking sheet and heat until melted. Remove sheet and place the Brussels sprouts and hazelnuts on it. Sprinkle with the salt and pepper. Roast for about 7 minutes. Sprinkle with water, toss, and continue to roast until tender and lightly browned (about 8 minutes more).

Candied Butternut Squash (6 servings)

1 large butternut squash (quartered lengthwise, seeds removed)
¼ cup melted butter
½ cup chopped pecans
¼ teaspoon ground cinnamon

Scoop the seeds out of the squash. Arrange squash, cut side down, in a baking dish. Pour in water to a depth of ¼ inch. Bake at 350°F until tender, 50 to 60 minutes. Cool, then peel. Cut into ½-inch slices, place in a baking dish, and top with the butter. Sprinkle with pecans and cinnamon. Bake an additional 20 minutes until glazed.

CONTINUED

DINNER 3, Cont.	**Dessert: Blueberries (6 servings)** 3 cups fresh blueberries whipped cream 1½ teaspoons cognac Top each serving with 1 teaspoon whipped cream and ¼ teaspoon cognac.

Nuts and seeds typically contain mono-unsaturated fats and are generally good sources of potassium and magnesium. They are calorie dense, so go lightly and choose from a variety including almonds, pistachios, walnuts, pecans and cashews. Sunflower, sesame and pumpkin are my favorite seeds. They may be eaten plain or included in salads and casseroles.

Day 4: 1889 calories (fat 1280, 68%; carb 400, 21%; protein 209, 11%)
Fat to carb ratio: 3.2:1

BREAKFAST 4	**Steel-Cut Coconut Oatmeal (1 serving)**
Calories 374 Fat 223 cal Carb 126 cal Protein 25 cal	¼ cup steel cut oatmeal 1 tablespoon dried goji berries 1 tablespoon quartered walnuts 1 tablespoon coconut oil ¼ Tsp cinnamon Place oats and goji berries in 1 cup of boiling water. Cook until smooth and let simmer for 10 minutes. Shortly before serving, add the coconut oil and then take off the heat and serve. Sprinkle with walnuts and cinnamon. Add some milk or half-and-half if desired.
LUNCH 4	**Greek Salad with Genoa Salami (4 servings)**
Calories 503 Fat 324 cal Carb 118 cal Protein 61 cal	1 tablespoon flax oil 6 tablespoons olive oil 3 tablespoons white wine vinegar 1 teaspoon dried oregano 1 clove garlic, minced 6 cups chopped romaine lettuce 1 can (15½ ounces) garbanzo beans, drained 1 red bell pepper, diced 1 red onion, sliced thinly 1 cup thinly sliced fresh fennel bulb ½ cup crumbled feta cheese 2 ounces Genoa salami, cut in strips ¼ cup pitted and sliced kalamata olives Whisk the oils, vinegar, oregano and garlic in a small bowl. Combine lettuce, garbanzo beans, bell pepper, red onion, fennel, feta cheese, salami and olives in a large bowl. Pour the dressing over the salad and toss. Place salad on platter and serve.

DINNER 4

Calories 1012
  Fat   733 cal
  Carb   156 cal
  Protein 123 cal

Macadamia Crusted Salmon (1 serving)
1 salmon steak (1 inch thick—6 ounces)
⅛ teaspoon salt
⅛ teaspoon coarsely ground pepper
1 egg white
¼ cup finely chopped Macadamia nuts
½ tablespoon olive oil
1 pat butter
1 tablespoon fresh minced parsley
½ teaspoon lemon juice

Sprinkle the fish with the salt and pepper. In a shallow bowl, whisk the egg white until frothy. Dip the fish in the egg white and gently pat the nut mixture into the fish. In a skillet, cook the fish in the olive oil over medium heat for 6 to 8 minutes on each side. Meanwhile, melt the butter and stir in the parsley and lemon juice. Drizzle over the fish and serve.

Curried Cabbage (1 serving)
1½ cups sliced cabbage
1½ pats butter
⅛ teaspoon mild curry powder
salt and pepper

Sauté the cabbage in the butter. Add the curry powder. Cover and cook until tender. Add salt and pepper to taste.

Sautéed Swiss Chard with Bacon (4 servings)
1 tablespoon olive oil
1 cup diced bacon
2 cloves garlic, smashed
1 pinch crushed red pepper flakes
1 pound Swiss chard, stems and leaves separated
½ cup vegetable stock
salt to taste

Coat a large sauce pan lightly with the olive oil and add the bacon, garlic and red pepper flakes. Bring to medium-high heat. When the garlic has turned light brown, remove and discard. At this point the bacon should be crispy. Add the Swiss chard stems and stock and cook until it is almost evaporated. Add the Swiss chard leaves and sauté until they are wilted. Season with salt and serve.

CONTINUED

DINNER 4, Cont.	**Dessert: Baked Vanilla Custard (1 serving)** 1 cup 2% milk 1 tablespoon sugar dash of salt 1 egg 1 egg white ⅜ teaspoon vanilla extract
	Combine milk, sugar, salt, egg, egg white, and vanilla extract and mix thoroughly. Pour into a custard cup. Place in pan of warm water and bake at 300°F for 1 hour.

Incorporate sources of the shorter-chain omega-3 fat α-linolenic acid, which occurs most abundantly in ground flax seeds or flax seed oil. It is also present in walnuts (or walnut oil), wheat germ, pumpkin seeds, spirulina, purslane, parsley, broccoli, kale, spinach, cabbage, dark green leafy vegetables and Brussels sprouts.

Day 5: 1978 calories (fat 1105, 56%; carb 562, 28%; protein 311, 16%)
Fat to carb ratio: 2.0:1

BREAKFAST 5 Calories 431 Fat 197 cal Carb 153 cal Protein 81 cal	**Country Breakfast (1 serving)** 2 poached eggs with salt and pepper 2 pieces bacon 1 slice of honeydew melon 1 slice Rye toast 1 pat butter 1 tablespoon strawberry jam
LUNCH 5 Calories 521 Fat 406 cal Carb 19 cal Protein 96 cal	**Zucchini Soup with Italian Sausage and Gouda Cheese (4 servings)** 2 tablespoons olive oil ¾ pound sweet Italian sausage 1 red onion, thinly sliced 3 medium fennel bulbs, halved, cored and thinly sliced 6 cups chicken stock 3 sprigs thyme 1 medium zucchini, thinly sliced 6 ounces Gouda cheese, finely shredded salt and pepper to taste Heat the olive oil in a saucepan. Add the sausage and cook over moderate heat until golden brown (about 10 minutes). Transfer to a plate. Add the onion to the saucepan and cook at moderate heat until slightly softened (about 4 minutes). Add the fennel, stock and thyme and cook until the fennel is very tender (about 45 minutes). Add the zucchini; cover and simmer about 2 minutes. Discard the thyme. Purée in a blender and return to the saucepan. Thinly slice the sausage and add it to the soup. Season with salt and pepper. Rewarm and then sprinkle with shredded cheese. Serve.
SNACK 5 Calories 424 Fat 215 cal Carb 116 cal Protein 93 cal	**(1 serving)** 2 ounces beef jerky 15 cashew nuts 4 dried apricots

DINNER 5	**Moroccan Dinner Stew (6 servings)**

Calories 602
Fat 287 cal
Carb 274 cal
Protein 41 cal
	2 tablespoons olive oil
	2 teaspoon butter
	1 onion, chopped coarsely
	2 cloves garlic, pressed (or more if you like)
	2 teaspoons turmeric
	2 teaspoons cumin seed
	1 teaspoon dill seed
	2 teaspoons coarsely ground black pepper
	½ teaspoon crushed red pepper
	1 pound ground beef
	2 cans (10 ounces each) whole tomatoes, with juice,
	   coarsely chopped
	8 cups low-sodium vegetable stock
	½ teaspoon salt
	2 cans (6 ounces each) garbanzo beans, drained
	½ cup golden raisins
	⅔ pound green beans, cut into 1-inch pieces
	1⅓ zucchini, quartered lengthwise and cut into 2-inch
	   pieces
	⅔ eggplant, skin on, coarsely chopped

Heat the olive oil and butter in a large skillet. Add the onion and sauté for 3 minutes. Add the garlic, turmeric, cumin, dill, and black and red pepper, and sauté 3 more minutes.

In a separate skillet, brown the ground beef, drain the fat and transfer to large slow cooker along with the tomatoes, vegetable stock, sautéed onion mixture and salt. Cover and cook on high for one hour.

Add the garbanzo beans, raisins, green beans, zucchini and eggplant. Turn the heat to low and continue cooking until the vegetables are tender, about 2½ more hours.

Dessert: Chilled Coconut Banana Mousse (6 servings)
6 ripe bananas
½ cup 2% milk
2 tablespoons coconut oil
big pinch of ground nutmeg
½ teaspoon vanilla extract

Peel bananas, place in a heavy freezer bag and freeze for 6 hours. Remove and cut each into 6 slices. Place into a food processor with the milk, coconut oil, nutmeg and vanilla extract. Process until creamy. Serve immediately.

Day 6: 2052 calories (fat 823, 56%; carb 562, 28%; protein 311, 16%)
Fat to carb ratio: 2.0:1

BREAKFAST 6 Calories 487 Fat　　148 cal Carb　　171 cal Protein 168 cal	**Smoked Salmon (Lox) and Cream Cheese (1 serving)** 4 ounces lox 1 ounce cream cheese 1 tablespoon 2% milk 4 tomato slices 2 mini-bagels, sliced in half capers 　Mix the cream cheese and milk. Spread on the lox. Place atop a tomato slice on a half mini-bagel. Sprinkle with several capers.
LUNCH 6 Calories 470 Fat　　155 cal Carb　　 86 cal Protein 229 cal	**Grilled Chicken Lettuce Wraps (2 wraps = 1 serving)** 4 ounces grilled chicken breast, sliced 1 cup diced tomato ½ cup diced cucumber ¼ cup shredded carrot 2 ounces Buttermilk Dressing (see below) 2 leaves lettuce 　Arrange the sliced chicken, tomato, cucumber and carrot on a large crisp leaf of lettuce. Drizzle with the dressing. Wrap up burrito style and serve with dill pickles. Makes 2 wraps. **Buttermilk Dressing** 3 tablespoons sour cream 3 tablespoons mayonnaise 2 tablespoon white wine vinegar ¼ cup buttermilk pepper to taste 　In a bowl, whisk the sour cream, mayonnaise and vinegar. Add the buttermilk and whisk. Season with pepper.
SNACK 6 Calories 393 Fat　　198 cal Carb　　121 cal Protein　 74 cal	**(1 serving)** 2 ounces provolone cheese 1 cup seedless green grapes 15 pistachio nuts

DINNER 6	**Cranberry Orange Pork tenderloin (6 servings)**

DINNER 6

Calories 702
Fat   322 cal
Carb   187 cal
Protein 193 cal

Cranberry Orange Pork tenderloin (6 servings)

2 pork tenderloins (about 1 pound each)
2 large cloves garlic
½ teaspoon ground cumin
½ teaspoon leaf thyme
½ teaspoon ground cinnamon
½ teaspoon ground allspice
pinch of ground cloves
1 tablespoon hazelnut oil
salt and pepper to taste
16 ounces fresh or frozen cranberries
1 can (12 ounces) mandarin orange slices in syrup
2 tablespoons sugar
juice and zest from 1 orange

Heat the oven to 425°F. Lightly oil a roasting pan. Trim excess fat off the pork.

Mash the garlic and blend with the cumin, thyme, cinnamon, allspice and cloves. Mix with 1 tablespoon of the hazelnut oil. Rub mixture over the pork. Place in oven and roast until the internal temperature is 155°F.

Meanwhile, in a saucepan combine the cranberries, mandarin orange slices and syrup, sugar, orange juice and zest and bring to a boil. Reduce heat and simmer for 8 to 10 minutes. Spoon some of the cranberry mixture over the pork and cook for 5 more minutes.

Heat the remaining cranberry mixture to serve with the sliced pork.

Let the pork stand for about 5 minutes before slicing.

CONTINUED

Don't forget coconut oil, which is the best cooking oil and a great source of energy because of its high content of medium-chain triglycerides (which also act as a powerful appetite suppressant).

DINNER 6, Cont.	**Jicama Cole Slaw (6 servings)** 1 head cabbage, shredded very thin 1 cup julienned green peppers 2 carrots, shredded 1 Bermuda onion, minced 1 cup sliced Jicama

Dressing
2 teaspoons sugar
1 teaspoon celery seed
1 teaspoon salt
¼ teaspoon black pepper
1 teaspoon dry mustard
1 teaspoon cilantro, minced
1 teaspoon fresh parsley
¼ teaspoon ground basil
½ cup macadamia nut oil
1 cup white balsamic vinegar

Combine the cabbage, pepper, minced onion and carrots. In a saucepan, combine all the dressing ingredients. Bring to a boil. Remove from the heat. While still hot, pour over the cabbage mixture, blending well. Cover and refrigerate for 8 hours or overnight. Add jicama and stir again just before serving.

Brussels Sprouts with Almonds and Pine Nuts (6 servings)
1 pound fresh Brussels sprouts
6 tablespoons butter
½ onion, chopped
salt and pepper to taste
1 tablespoon freshly squeezed lemon juice
¼ cup toasted slivered almonds
¼ cup toasted pine nuts

Boil the Brussels sprouts in water until just tender, 3 to 4 minutes. Split one open to see if it is cooked in the center. Strain and place in ice water to preserve color. Cut into halves.

Sauté the onion in 2–3 tablespoons of the butter until translucent. Add the Brussels sprouts to the remaining butter. Cook over medium heat for several more minutes. Add salt and pepper. Don't overcook or the sprouts will become bitter.

Remove from heat. Toss in half of the almonds and all the pine nuts and lemon juice. Place in a serving dish. Garnish with the rest of the almonds.

CONTINUED

DINNER 6, Cont.	**Dessert: Chocolate and Raspberries (1 serving)** 2 squares dark chocolate (1 inch on a side) 10 red raspberries

Remember two things: 1) that the brain, which is made of fat, requires a continuous supply of healthy fatty nutrients in the diet to keep it functioning properly, and 2) that over the past 30 to 40 years during the low-fat eating experiment, obesity and diabetes have become commonplace. If eating less fat has contributed to this disastrous situation, eating more of the right type of fat should certainly help.

Day 7: 2037 calories (fat 981, 48%; carb 600, 30%; protein 456, 22%)
Fat to carb ratio: 1.6:1

BREAKFAST 7	Simple Banana Almond Smoothie (1 serving)
Calories 488 Fat 161 cal Carb 135 cal Protein 192 cal	¼ cup almonds 1 tablespoon flax oil 1 ripe banana 30 grams whey protein 1 cup soy milk ½–1 cup ice cubes Mix all ingredients in a blender and blend well. Enjoy immediately!
LUNCH 7	The Best Egg Salad Sandwich Ever! (4 servings)
Calories 431 Fat 222 cal Carb 142 cal Protein 67 cal	6 large eggs 1½ tablespoons mayonnaise salt and pepper to taste ¼ teaspoon lemon juice ½ bunch chives, chopped 2 celery ribs, washed and finely chopped 8 leaves romaine lettuce 8 slices whole grain toast Creating the best egg salad sandwich requires properly boiling the egg. It must be boiled so that the center sets yet stays moist. Then, dunk the egg in a bowl of ice water immediately to stop the cooking. Place the eggs in a pot and cover with cold water by ½ inch. Bring to a gentle boil. Turn off the heat, cover, and let sit for exactly 7 minutes. Have a big bowl of ice water ready when the eggs are done cooking and place them in the ice bath for 3 minutes to stop the cooking. Crack and peel each egg and place in a mixing bowl. Add the mayonnaise and some salt and pepper and mash with a fork. Don't overdo it. Stir in the celery and chives. To assemble each sandwich: place the lettuce on a piece of toast, top with the egg salad mixture and finish by covering with the second piece of toast. Enjoy with ⅓ avocado, sliced and 1 ripe plum.

DINNER 7
 	
Calories 1118
  Fat   981 cal
  Carb   600 cal
  Protein 197 cal
	Scallops with Endive (serves 2)
	¼ cup extra-virgin olive oil
	juice of 1 lemon
	salt and pepper to taste
	2 ounces almond oil
	10 endive leaves
	10 large scallops
	1 tablespoon chopped fresh chives
	1 tablespoon finely diced tomatoes

In a small mixing bowl, combine the olive oil, lemon juice, salt and pepper. Whisk together to make the dressing. Set aside.

Heat a sauté pan and coat with the almond oil. Sauté the endive leaves until golden brown. Remove from the pan. Arrange 5 endive leaves on each plate in a star pattern.

Add the scallops to the pan and sauté until they are golden brown. Add salt and pepper. Remove from pan and place 4 in the center of each endive star. Place the fifth on top in the center. Drizzle 1½ tablespoons of the dressing over the scallops and along the leaves. Sprinkle the chopped chives and diced tomatoes over the leaves and serve immediately.

Spinach Mousse (serves 4)
1 pound fresh spinach
3 egg whites
⅛ teaspoon nutmeg
⅛ teaspoon salt
⅛ teaspoon pepper
2 ounces heavy cream

Blanche the spinach for 30 seconds, then dry thoroughly. Place in a blender with the egg whites, nutmeg, salt and pepper. Blend for about a minute. Drizzle in the cream and continue blending. Chill for several hours until ready to serve.

CONTINUED

DINNER 7, Cont.	**Peppers with Orzo and Mint (6 servings)** 1 can (28 ounces) Italian tomatoes 2 zucchini, grated ½ cup chopped fresh mint leaves ½ cup grated Romano cheese ¼ cup extra-virgin olive oil 3 cloves garlic, minced 1 teaspoon salt 1 teaspoon freshly ground black pepper 4 cups chicken broth 1 cup orzo 6 green peppers

	Heat the oven to 400°F. Pour the tomatoes into a large bowl and break apart. Add the zucchini, mint, olive oil, garlic, salt and pepper. Stir together.
	   In a medium saucepan, bring the chicken broth to a boil over high heat. Add the orzo and cook for 4 minutes. Transfer the orzo to the large bowl with the tomato mixture. Transfer the chicken broth left behind to a 3-quart baking dish.
	   Slice the tops off the peppers and remove all the ribs and seeds. Place the peppers in the baking dish with the warm chicken broth. Spoon the orzo mixture into the peppers. Cover with foil and bake for 45 minutes. Remove the foil, sprinkle with the grated cheese and bake until the cheese is golden brown (about 15 more minutes). Remove and transfer to a serving plate.

CONTINUED

Blend color into the diet by selecting fruits and veggies in all hues of the rainbow. Be sure to mix and match because different colors provide different nutrients.

DINNER 7, Cont.	Dessert: Apricot Ambrosia (serves 6)
	1 can (15 ounces) apricot halves, drained
	1 tablespoon coconut oil
	3 ounces sweetened condensed milk
	2⅔ tablespoons lemon juice
	4 ounces crushed pineapple
	¼ cup slivered almonds
	½ cup whipped cream
	½ cup flaked coconut, toasted
	Chop 6 apricot halves for a garnish. Set aside. In a blender, purée the remaining apricots and coconut oil.
	In a large bowl, combine the condensed milk, lemon juice, pineapple and puréed apricot mixture. Fold in the almonds and whipped cream.
	In each individual serving dish, place 2 teaspoons of toasted coconut and then ½ cup of the apricot mixture. Top with the apricot garnish and 2 teaspoons of toasted coconut. Chill and serve cold.

The total nutritional information for the week (average per day) is

Calories	1942
Fat	1031 calories (53%)
Carb	513 calories (26%)
Protein	398 calories (21%)

Fat to carb ratio 2.0:1

These recipes are provided as examples of meals that are possible to include in this way of eating. They are to be used as guidelines and jumping off points for the universe of potential food combinations that should be limited only by your imagination.

The caloric content provided by the meal plans listed above isn't appropriate for everyone. Again, it is merely illustrative because 1,942 calories a day may be too many or not enough for different individuals. I have included an equation below for determining an estimate of your daily caloric requirements.

The BMR (basal metabolic rate) is the number of calories your body consumes to keep you alive in the resting state and it must be adjusted based on activity level. I have provided typical activities to help determine your PAR (physical activity ratio) for the day. To roughly approximate your total daily caloric requirement you must multiply the BMR by the PAR.

Total Caloric Requirement = BMR x PAR

CALCULATING BMR

BMR = 4.54 (W) + 16.88(H) – 4.92(A)

Where: W = Weight in pounds
H = Height in inches
A = Age in years

Note: Men must add 5 to the total. Women must subtract 161.

CALCULATING PAR

PAR	Type of activity
1.0 – 1.4	Sitting quietly, watching TV, writing, playing cards, listening to music
1.5 – 1.8	Sewing, driving, ironing, light office work, using the computer
1.9 – 2.4	Easy household chores, cooking, cleaning, dusting, washing
2.5 – 3.3	Dressing, showering, vacuuming, making beds, painting, operating tools
3.4 – 4.4	Mopping the floor, gardening, cleaning windows, moderate walking, playing golf, carpentry work
4.5 – 4.9	Chopping wood, brisk walking, dancing, moderate swimming, cycling, jogging, digging, shoveling
6.0 – 7.9	Very brisk walking, cross country skiing, stair climbing, moderate jogging or cycling, tennis, heavy swimming

To calculate your average daily PAR you must determine how many hours of the day you do certain activities and assign each activity a PAR value. Then multiply the PAR value by the fraction of the day it is performed and add them all up as shown below.

◊ Assume you sleep for 9 hours a day. (PAR = 1)

◊ You exercise vigorously for 1 hour a day (PAR = 7)

◊ You perform light office work for 8 hours. (PAR = 1.7)

◊ You perform housework for 2 hours. (PAR = 2.1)

◊ You spend 1 hour showering, dressing, making the bed, etc. (PAR = 2.7)

◊ You do 2 hours of computer work at home. (PAR = 1.5)

◊ You watch TV for 1 hour. (PAR = 1.1)

These activities total 24 hours—a complete day. To determine your average PAR, calculate what fraction of the day (for example 1/24, 8/24 and so on) you do each avtivity and add them all up as follows: (9/24) x 1 + (1/24) x 7 + (8/24) x 1.7 + (2/24) x 2.1 + (1/24) x 2.7 + (2/24) x 1.5 + (1/24) x 1.1 = 1.69. So your average PAR over the course of the day (24 hours) is 1.69.

To calculate your total caloric requirement, multiply that number by your BMR. If you are a 50-year-old female who weighs 155 pounds and is 5'5" tall, your BMR is calculated as: (4.54 x 155) + (16.88 x 65) – (4.92 x 50) – 161 which turns out to be 1,394 calories. To calculate your total caloric requirement just multiply that by your PAR of 1.69 and you arrive at 2,356 calories. If you had been more sedentary with a PAR of 1.4 your total energy requirement would have been just 1,952 calories. These calculations provide a very rough estimate of the total number of calories you would need to eat to remain weight stable.

My Favorite Snack

As a special treat, my favorite snack is Heather's spicy mixed nuts recipe. I have these around to munch on when I get hungry.

SNACK	Heather's Spicy Mixed Nuts

Serving size: 16–18 nuts
 	
Calories   162
  Fat   120 cal
  Carb   21 cal
  Protein   21 cal
  Fat to carb
  ratio: 6:1
	1 egg white
	1 tablespoon water
	4 cups mixed nuts (equally divided between almonds, pecan halves, walnut halves)
	2 tablespoons sugar
	1 teaspoon salt
	1½ teaspoon ground cumin
	1 teaspoon paprika
	¼ teaspoon ground ginger
	2 teaspoons cinnamon
	1 teaspoon nutmeg
	
	Preheat oven to 300°F. In a mixing bowl, beat the egg white and water until frothy. Add the nuts and toss until well coated. Transfer to a wire mesh sieve and drain for 5 minutes.
	Meanwhile, in a large plastic bag combine the sugar, salt, cumin, paprika, ginger, cinnamon and nutmeg. Add the nuts and shake well to coat with the spices.
	Spread evenly on an ungreased 15-by-10-by-1 inch baking pan. Bake until the nuts are toasted, stirring every 10 minutes (35 to 40 minutes).
	Remove from the oven and transfer to a foil sheet.

Note: In all of the nutritional information I have provided, I have used the "effective" carb concept, which means subtracting out the carbs that fall under fiber from the total carb content:

Effective Carbs = Total Carb Content – Fiber Carb Content

Beverages

Green and black tea or water with lemon are my favorites. On a hot day a tall glass of iced tea is lovely. White or red wine with dinner is nice if it fits your palate.

• • •

You should use these recipes as guidelines to configure your own delicacies. Just remember to be creative; use plenty of herbs and spices; add color to each dish; and explore foods you haven't tried before. Make eating a special time of the day—one you prepare for and one you truly enjoy!

7

Move It to Lose It

Getting in touch with your body is very important especially when you are trying to lose weight. Emotional eating must be distinguished from true hunger, and boredom from starvation. Subtle alterations in body composition develop and must be recognized. Being physically active enhances our ability to detect each of these changes.

We were born to move, to be active and to challenge our bodies. For this reason it is necessary to incorporate into our daily lives activities that elevate heart rate, stretch our muscles and produce all the beneficial hormonal changes that make losing weight much easier. All of these things are great for the brain and the body...and they just plain feel good once you get used to them!

It is no surprise that being active on a regular basis is part of a healthy lifestyle. And to reap the benefits you don't have to be Michael Phelps. Setting aside the time and sticking to it are what really count—hence the Nike slogan *Just Do It*. After each session you will feel more energized than you did after the previous one. Although most of us can begin moving in a safe fashion, it is best to get a doctor's OK before starting any exercise program.

A Big Waste of Time?

To properly evaluate the benefits of the Feed Your Brain Lose Your Belly diet and activity program, we tested it in a group of human volunteers. You will be hearing about the results in

Chapter 11. I refer to the subjects who lost weight on the program as our *Biggest Losers*. When they began the activity part of the program, several of them thought it was going to take a lot of time—time they didn't have to spare. Yet, by the end of the study those who most ardently resisted the activity program became its staunchest supporters. What brought about this change of heart?

If you haven't done anything in a while to break a sweat, it can be surprising how winded you become just from walking up a flight of stairs. That's why it makes sense to start slowly, pace yourself and be comfortable. Otherwise, you might get hurt. When this happens, any activity or exercise program comes to a screeching halt. So, it is better to be the tortoise rather than the hare in this situation, which also helps to ensure that you understand and feel good about your increased level of physical activity. Stressing this approach during the weekly meetings with the volunteers who were on the program helped remove any anxiety about exercising.

The other recommendation we heard repeatedly was that to facilitate compliance, simplicity and convenience were of paramount importance. Another recommendation was to choose a friend with whom you can exercise (an "exercise buddy" to help keep you on the program), compare notes and just plain enjoy the experience. This will help keep you on track no matter what the weather is like.

When approached in this manner, working out soon becomes something to look forward to. Believe it or not, you might even start to feel cheated if you miss a few sessions. It can even help

Start slowly, pace yourself and be comfortable.

with sleep difficulties—both falling asleep and being able to sleep through the night. You'll feel rejuvenated after you get your blood pumping. And stairs will gradually become less of a challenge.

It was for all these reasons that almost everyone felt that including some physical activity in their daily schedule was vital. It also became a personal challenge—with all of the participants pushing themselves to surpass what they had accomplished the prior week. This was easy to measure because all were given pedometers to wear, and they graphed the number of steps they took every day. A few of our experts were startled to learn how far one can walk without going outdoors—even though getting fresh air was so stimulating.

Keep It Simple

Walking was the preferred form of activity in the clinical study. It doesn't require a pool, track or treadmill. Plus, it starts as soon as you step out the front door, so no gym pass is necessary. The local shopping mall was a favorite venue because it was enclosed, which assured protection from the elements. It provided a safe and well-lit place to walk while also being a great place for people watching. Since we attempted to make our activity program as user friendly as possible, this was a perfect solution because it allowed everyone to participate and enjoy it.

What seemed to work best was walking three times a week on alternating days (such as Monday, Wednesday and Friday) for 30 to 50 minutes. Each session included a ten-minute warm-up and a similar ten-minute cool-down period at the end. Almost everyone started at 30 minutes and slowly extended their time to 45 or 50 minutes. Please note that if you have other health problems or haven't exercised in a while, you may need to start more slowly. If so, don't be discouraged because you'll be surprised at how quickly you will be able to increase your exercise time as your body becomes accustomed to the exertion and you start to lose weight.

The warm-up and cool-down periods consisted of slower intervals designed to get the blood pumping and make sure there were no injuries. The main exercise segment consisted of a period lasting 10 to 30 minutes depending on where people were in the program.

During this segment the volunteers used one of three approaches. (1) Each time they walked they increased their speed slightly compared to what it had been during the prior session but never to exceed the threshold that made it uncomfortable to carry on a conversation with a walking partner. (2) Others used a different approach consisting of intervals of faster walking (for 2 to 5 minutes) alternating with slower intervals. (3) Another method employed (during an individual session) was walking at a slowly increasing rate in a crescendo fashion to a peak speed, followed by a decrescendo back down to the rate at which the person had started. All of these approaches are fine. Using one method and then another is also acceptable. It is important to mix up any workout regimen to keep it lively. What we stressed was getting into the habit of being active and making it a part of the daily routine—preferably with a friend. All study participants wore their pedometers and kept track of the number of steps they took during their walks. These were subsequently entered into their Log Book.

The second component of the activity program involved light resistance training (working out with weights) around the home. This made it simple for everyone. Easily held household objects weighing from 1 to 20 pounds were identified. They became the "weights" that were hoisted several times a week. Bags of coffee, cans of soup or soda, 5-pound bags of flour, sacks of wild bird seed and plastic gallon water containers were easy to locate. Gallon containers are particularly useful because the amount of liquid in them can easily be increased as muscle endurance improves. Some items were held in one hand while others required a double-handed grip. Light weights were used initially.

As people became stronger they progressed to somewhat heavier weights. No weights were necessary for some of the other muscle building exercises. Upper body, lower body and trunk workouts were alternated throughout the week. Weight training was usually performed for 20 minutes every Tuesday and Thursday.

At this time it will be helpful to take a moment to go over some terminology that you might not be familiar with. Imagine that you are holding a can of soup in your right hand. A *repetition* is the act of moving the can through a full range of motion of any particular joint—in this case, the elbow. A group of repetitions performed sequentially, usually 6 to 10, is called a *set*. Usually two sets of any specified exercise were performed for each of three muscle groups. This simple approach takes about 20 minutes to complete.

Let's walk through a typical session. We'll start with arm and shoulder exercises including the *deltoid* muscle, the *biceps* muscle and the *triceps* muscle. The biceps is the muscle that bends the elbow joint in an upward manner. Its range of motion begins starting with the arm hanging in a resting position nearly straight down. A can of soup or something slightly heavier is held in the hand. Start bending the elbow up until your hand is near your ear where the motion ends before being reversed—which means *slowly* lowering your arm until the elbow is almost straight again. The full cycle of motion constitutes one repetition. It is usually

repetition (rep) =
moving through a full
range of motion of a joint

set =
a group of repetitions

repeated *slowly* 6 to 10 times. This collection of repetitions is called a set. A moment later the same 6 to 10 repetitions are repeated. These are usually shortened to "reps" and "sets." The other arm is then put through the same group of movements. This completes the workout for the biceps muscles.

The deltoid is the muscle that moves the shoulder. When you place your hand on the shoulder, you are feeling the deltoid muscle. With your hand at your side using the same can you just used (keeping the arm straight), *slowly* raise the hand through an arc out to the side until it is parallel to the ground. You will have moved your hand through a 90-degree arc. Now *slowly* reverse this motion. That completes one rep. Repeat this movement 6 to 10 times and stop. A moment later, repeat the same number of reps. Perform the same exercises on the other arm. Now you have completed two muscles.

The third muscle is the triceps muscle. It straightens (or extends) the elbow joint. For this exercise you will need a heavier can such as a large juice can. Grasp it in both hands holding it over your head with your arms straight up. Now bend both elbows 90 degrees by lowering the can behind your head, pause, then straighten them again over the head. This is one rep. Repeat 6 to 10 times to complete one set of triceps exercises. After you are rested, repeat the set. This ends the upper body strength training session. It will take about twenty minutes to complete. The same time will be required for the lower body and trunk sessions. Weight training is an intense form of exercise. If you have never done anything like it, you might consider seeking help from a certified trainer or an experienced friend. As you become stronger you will need to use slightly heavier weights.

Suggested leg exercises include knee extension, knee flexion and ankle extension. For the ankle extension training, the calf muscle is exercised. Grasp a plastic one-gallon water container in each hand. Start with them only half filled. In a comfortable standing position start by rocking up onto your toes, hold that for two seconds, then roll back down onto the soles of your feet. This constitutes one rep. Repeat it 6 to 10 times, wait a minute or two, then do a second set.

For the *quadriceps* muscle (the "quad" or the thigh muscle), lunges are a good way to build up strength. When getting started I would suggest not holding any weights the first several times. Try to perform a series of lunges, first on the left side then the right. Start in a comfortable standing position with your feet side by side. While keeping your back upright, take one step forward. As you do, lower your pelvis until your front knee is bent almost 90 degrees then hold this position for 1 to 3 seconds. Straighten up, take the next step and repeat the maneuver on the other leg. Repeat 6 times. This constitutes one set. If you are comfortable continuing, try another set.

Knee flexion exercises the *hamstring* muscles. An easy way to strengthen them is by sitting on the edge of an easy chair. Sit up straight with your feet on the ground and your heels touching the chair. Starting with one foot, press and hold your heel firmly against the front of the chair. Hold this position for 4 or 5 seconds, then relax. Repeat 6 to 10 times with the same foot. Now perform the same series using the other foot. If you can comfortably repeat another set, do so. This completes the lower extremity strength training.

Trunk training typically strengthens your side, abdomen and back muscles. Starting in a comfortable standing position with your feet about 12 inches apart, place your hands on your hips. This is the neutral position for the three trunk exercises below. For the sides, slowly lower one shoulder laterally to about a 45-degree angle. Hold it for three seconds then perform the same maneuver in the opposite direction. This constitutes one rep. Perform 6 to 10 reps, then repeat the set.

Starting from the same neutral standing position described above with your hands on your hips, bend forward about 45 degrees. You will feel the muscles in your back tighten. Hold this position for three seconds then slowly straighten up. This constitutes one rep. Perform 6 to 10 reps. After a brief rest, repeat the set.

For the abdominal muscles, start upright in the neutral position. Then lean backward 20 to 30 degrees until you can feel your abdominal muscles tighten. Hold that position for three seconds then return to neutral. That is one rep. As above, repeat 6 to 10 times. This is one set. After a brief rest, repeat the set. This completes the trunk exercises.

It is important to do all of the exercises slowly to gain full advantage of the challenge presented by each motion. Doing them rapidly creates momentum that reduces the difficulty of each exercise. If it is too difficult to do an exercise slowly, lighten the weight until you become stronger and can increase it again.

When you have become comfortable with these exercises you can begin to include others. There are many web sites and other exercise guides you can use to become more adept at weight training. I also suggest joining a gym and working with a qualified trainer.

The third component of the exercise program incorporates activities that improve balance and coordination. Examples include walking on irregular paths, jumping rope, playing ping-pong and hopping first on one foot then the other. Although these activities don't sound very difficult, everyone felt they were important. I

The Feed Your Brain,
Lose Your Belly Exercise Program
• Walking •
• Resistance (weight) training •
• Improving balance and
coordination •

believe they also help prevent injuries by improving balance skills. They can be practiced separately or performed while walking.

The Feed Your Brain Lose Your Belly exercise program includes all three types of activity. Walking should be performed three times a week for 30 to 50 minutes—usually on Monday, Wednesday and Friday. The weight training is done twice a week on alternate days and usually takes twenty to thirty minutes. Approximately 10 minutes of balance and agility activities can be scheduled whenever time allows, typically several times per week.

We recommended that study volunteers perform resistance training twice a week, usually on Tuesday and Thursday. They rotated the three body areas sequentially as follows: 1) upper body strengthening, 2) trunk activity and 3) lower body muscle groups. We were not attempting to make people muscle-bound. The goal was to include some "power" training (weight training) that augmented the aerobic benefits of walking. It is also great for bone health.

Just like they recorded what they ate, every workout was documented by detailing what was done in a personal Log Book. It also allowed each subject to track their progress.

Don't Overdo It!

The study subjects were counseled to adhere to the activity program but to stay within their comfort zone. This approach was recommended for three reasons—to avoid injuries, to make it easier to stick with the program and to keep it fun.

We suggested levels of activity that were "mild" to "moderate" because we wanted everyone to be comfortable and to have a stable foundation from which to build. We were hoping they would achieve a sense of well-being, an improvement in cardiovascular fitness and enhanced strength and balance...*all without stimulating appetite excessively*.

Additional Benefits

As was mentioned previously, the mere sight of someone wearing a pedometer generated support from coworkers, friends and relatives, which made it easier to stick with the program. It also created new friends and walking partners for a number of our volunteers. These were welcome and unexpected perks of wearing that funny little box around wherever they went. It was like a "yellow badge of courage."

Positive Feedback

This approach to exercise and activity was enthusiastically supported by everyone. It made them all feel better both mentally and physically, helped burn calories and created an esprit de corps among the group. The recommendations were the same for each participant. However, they were personalized and adapted to accommodate various schedules and routines. Each of the volunteers felt that this was a fun and useful part of the program and enthusiastically suggested that you incorporate a similar version in your activity regimen. Much to their surprise, by the conclusion of the clinical trial many of the participants had progressed sufficiently to take the next step and join a gym or recreation center for exposure to a greater variety of aerobic and resistance machines. An unexpected benefit of the "move it to lose it" program was the increased zest for life that was engendered. Hopefully, you'll experience that as well!

Part 3

Training Your Brain to Lose Your Belly

8
How It Feels to Gain Weight

Ten years ago, one in four Americans was obese. Now that number is one in three! On average, being obese usually means being about 25 pounds beyond just being overweight. So, if you are a middle-aged female who is about 5 feet, 5 inches and your ideal weight is 125 pounds, if you weigh 150 pounds you meet the criteria for being overweight. If you weigh 175 pounds, you are considered obese! About one-third of the weight of people who fall into this category is fat tissue!

This means they are carrying around almost *60 pounds of fat*—upstairs, downstairs, while working and even when exercising. No wonder it takes a toll on our bodies and joints. Imagine carrying a 60-pound pack everywhere you go. If you were short of breath, it wouldn't be surprising. But that is exactly what many of us are doing. More than 90 million Americans are obese and 180 million are overweight.

Carrying excess weight is also associated with an array of serious health issues including diabetes, high blood pressure, stroke, heart attack, heart failure, certain types of cancer, gallstones, gout, osteoarthritis and sleep apnea. As if those aren't frightening enough, we can now add memory loss and Alzheimer's disease to this daunting list. Needless to say, accumulation of body fat is a huge and growing problem!

In addition to taking a toll on us personally, the fiscal burden it imposes on the country's health care budget is staggering. Annual health costs attributed to being overweight currently exceed $100 billion. This represents almost 10 percent of the total medical spending in this country. There are even current predictions suggesting that most Americans will be overweight within the next ten years!

With figures (and figures) like these, one might think there is something in the drinking water. Perhaps that is true. But there is *definitely* something in the food we eat. While genes clearly may predispose certain individuals to excessive energy storage (meaning fat storage), the emergence of widespread obesity has only recently become a problem. Surprisingly, not too long ago starvation was a much more pressing concern than obesity.

Why is it so easy to gain weight? Why is it so difficult to lose weight? And why is gaining weight so difficult to deal with? To help shed light on these important issues we have interviewed a number of "experts" in weight loss as defined by the amount of weight (and fat) they were able to shed (and are still losing) during the clinical trial in which they participated. They are our "Biggest Losers!" Because they know how important it is, they gladly took the time to talk about why they gained weight, how it made them feel and what helped them during their weight loss journey.

To maintain confidentiality, I have not included their real names. However, their emotional commitment is evident when you hear what they say about how becoming overweight affected their lives. They want to get the message out to anyone and everyone who has a weight problem, has attempted and failed to lose weight previously or would like to embark on a new thinner, healthier and happier lifestyle. Our heroes are here for you and are

More than 90 million Americans are obese and 180 million are overweight.

ready to reveal their highs and lows along with the desperate times and inspirational insights that made them successful. So let's hear what they have to say!

Gaining Weight—Personal Stories

For many of our experts, carrying a few (or many) extra pounds has been a life-long problem. Emily H described her mother's heartbreak at not having a daughter she could enter in a beauty pageant. School was a nightmare. Kids can be cruel, which for her was an ongoing source of agony. When she entered college, the so-called "freshman fifteen" turned out to be thirty. After graduation things only became worse and because of her weight gain getting a job was difficult. Pregnancy was another step in the journey that culminated with her breaking the 280-pound plateau. She was even beginning to feel like she would never see her feet again. To make matters worse, diabetes and hypertension developed. Her dad had died of a stroke and it was beginning to look like she would be the next in line. Emily even suffered recurring fears about not being there for her son as he grew up.

Michelle D knew from personal experience what it meant to live a yo-yo life and had become an experienced yo-yo dieter. Losing weight when she was younger had been fairly easy. But then she would gain it all back. With each ensuing cycle it became harder and harder to return to her baseline weight. Maternity clothes were making their way into her closet and were replacing the fashionable styles she had become used to wearing. After several yo-yo periods she sensed she was losing the battle of the bulge. Her life seemed to be spinning out of control and she even began experiencing panic attacks.

Emma T's downfall appeared to be travel. Regardless of whether it was for business or pleasure, she always seemed to come home a little heavier. Entertaining clients often meant lavish dinners, wine and desserts—items in which she didn't normally indulge. Who knew what was in the sauces? Portions were also larger than those she served at home. To make matters worse, she liked to eat as did her friends.

Subconsciously, they seemed to encourage each other. What started as a dessert "for the table" often turned into three or four desserts. And after dinner drinks were frequently followed by fancy coffee creations. She traveled at least twice a month, so over time the dinners (and pounds) added up. Because business activities were such a big part of her life, Emma was conflicted about remaining "part of the group" while knowing that this lifestyle was contributing to her weight gain.

Another work-related diet breaker is stress. Dottie G loved her job but soon learned that working for her boss was not easy. Her performance never seemed to be quite good enough. According to her supervisor she needed too much guidance, couldn't think on her own, didn't problem solve very effectively and maybe just had some bad luck thrown in.

Because she has a special needs daughter and depends on performance bonuses to make ends meet, Dottie found herself stretched fairly thin when they didn't materialize. To help alleviate the internal turmoil the work environment created, she found solace in foods she knew were not healthy such as chocolate covered almonds, Oreos and jellybeans. She unsuccessfully attempted to parse them out during the day. Despite her best efforts the bags were usually empty when she got home. In her situation stress was a real diet killer. Feeling overwhelmed had become the norm for Dottie.

Being born large—10 pounds and 6 ounces in her case—is not uncommon in Darcy N's family because her mom is diabetic. Her two older sisters started out big and stayed that way. They were both at least fifty pounds overweight and had large kids, too.

Stress can be a diet-breaker.

What made things even worse, Darcy seemed to eat like a bird. She claimed that whatever she ate went directly to her thighs and "stuck like glue." Her friends agreed that if anyone was inclined to gain weight it was poor Darcy. This perception is now gaining support in the medical literature based largely on the insulin-obesity connection.

Jim B's situation is a bit different. He was the youngest child in a family of eleven and can't recall a time when money hadn't been a problem. He doesn't know who his father is and his mother wasn't around very often. He felt lucky to have a sister, Linda, who made sure he had his lunch money, got to school on time and made it home safely at the end of the day. Dinner was usually some sort of fast food, which is what he had become accustomed to. He ate whatever was put in front of him and had no sense of what is considered to be good or bad food.

Now he is in his mid-forties and is working as a janitor at the local high school. His diet hasn't changed. While not excessively heavy, he has developed Type 2 diabetes and is on medication to treat it. Recently, one of his friends suggested he take a course in nutrition at the local community college. He now wants to get off the medicine he is taking and believes he can accomplish that goal if he loses weight.

Kat R, short for Katrina, grew up in an abusive family. It seemed like whatever she did was never good enough—her grades were inadequate; sports performance was not up to par; her room was never clean enough; her bed was never made right and her closets were too messy. In other words nothing she did was ever up to expectations. She doesn't remember ever receiving a compliment from her parents, and she subsequently (probably subconsciously) married a man who shared many of her father's traits.

For her food was more a nutrient for the soul than for the body. It was a reward for what she achieved at work, a comfort for what she didn't and punishment for not meeting her own goals. For as long as she could recall she had considered herself to be an "emotional eater." She received gratification from food because it was the only positive factor in her life. Unfortunately for her, it contributed to her yearly ten to fifteen pound weight gain—adding an unwieldy 61 pounds to her petite frame over five years.

Chantal W ate whenever she became bored, which was not uncommon. Working at home, when her mind wandered she got up, went to the pantry and grabbed a handful of chips, crackers or whatever else was available.

As you know, there are many different approaches to eating and just as many reasons to gain weight and keep it on. In addition to these insights, it is not difficult to imagine many other reasons for finding yourself becoming pudgy. And as we have seen, the weight itself is frequently not the only thing that needs to be dealt with, or even the worst thing, because of the secondary psychological and emotional fallout it creates.

Overweight (Again)!

How it feels to be overweight is never good, but it seems to affect us all quite differently and produces a variable array of responses. It might even generate different feelings at different times in one's life, depending on the situation and history of past experiences. Trudy K referred to her weight gain as an indication of inadequacy. She said if she was unable to control what she put in her mouth, there was not much hope of successfully controlling anything else. It was as if gaining weight was a metaphor for many of the failures she had suffered over the years—a different manifestation of the same "underlying pathology."

Deb K first realized she was too heavy when she was a teenager. It was at about the same time that her complexion flared up. At first she was unsure of whether the problem was due to stress, boys or weight gain—or maybe a combination of all three. But weight was clearly a factor. She later became aware of the social impact of being heavy when she was ridiculed by her classmates and had trouble getting dates. As she gained more

*Weight gain may not be
the only problem you need to deal
with in your life*

weight, she soon realized that finding clothes that fit and looked attractive was difficult, so she started wearing looser tops that hung out over her pants in a futile attempt to hide her excess pounds.

Later in life she began to have shortness of breath when she walked up more than one flight of stairs. She questioned her doctor about this. He explained that it was because she was carrying around 50 extra pounds and asked her to imagine how she would feel if she had to tote the equivalent of two heavy shopping bags wherever she went.

That's when it dawned on her that being overweight could have potentially serious health ramifications. She was well aware that her dad, who had been quite heavy for a long time, had died of a heart attack.

The other thing that really bothered her was that she found it was impossible to do many things that she had been able to do previously, such as playing tennis and skiing. Her body was failing her! Almost uniformly our experts noted that as they gained weight, they tired much more easily, running out of energy without exerting themselves or doing anything very strenuous.

Todd D and Marie L said the thing that bothered them the most was the way they felt in their clothes—like stuffed sausages. Several others hated the way their bodies seemed to jiggle when they walked—a perception they were painfully aware of. Each movement was an ominous indicator of these changes.

Possibly the most poignant reminder of the impact of gaining weight was the realization of the associated health issues and the attendant fragility of life. The potential consequences of these insights made each and every weight loss expert in the study reflect upon the fact that they might not be there to take care of their aging parents or growing children. This single observation was the most prescient and motivating factor that kept them on the program.

What You Need to Know

If you look around, the first thing that should strike you is that *you are not alone!* No matter how out of shape, overweight or depressed you are about being too heavy, there are many others who are in worse shape and need to lose weight even more urgently than you do. You should also acknowledge that losing weight might not be easy for you. However, I suggest you keep in mind the fact that many people have walked in your shoes and a number of them *have* achieved their goals! While success is a great motivator, there will be times when, regardless of what you do, you find yourself stuck on a dreaded weight loss plateau. This produces many negative reactions including desperation, anxiety, depression and fear of failure.

Our Biggest Losers have been there and felt that. What they want you to know is that you CAN do it. They are painfully aware of how it feels to step on the scale only to be confronted with no weight loss or even worse—weight gain. Since the best time to weigh yourself is in the morning, news like that can set a very poor tone for the day. As a matter of fact, starting off with such unwelcome news probably won't lead to a very happy day. Nonetheless, you must persevere.

Our weight loss experts will be by your side every step of the way, giving you the same type of assistance they needed while they were going through the process. Just like pitchers and batters must change subtle aspects of their approach to baseball based on how things are going, so must you. That is a key component of any successful strategy. Remember, you have a built in knowledgeable and dedicated support system committed to your success—our "Biggest Losers."

Based on what worked for them, we have compiled inspirational, practical and easy to follow tips for success. Our experts hope that their useful pointers will help you lose weight and maintain your sanity. The recommendations they provide are not cast in stone to be followed without variation, but instead are guidelines that are to be personalized to meet your needs, situation and outlook. Remaining dedicated while dealing with a complicated lifestyle can be exceedingly difficult. Armed with the tips for success you will be reading about, we are certain you will become a Big Loser as well! The inspirational observations and guidelines of our study participants will help you to remain committed and understand what your body will be encountering as you embark on your weight loss journey. These insights will enable you to be successful and to help others achieve their goals as well!

You know yourself better than anyone else. Are you up for the challenge?

9
Pearls of Wisdom from the Experts

As you get started you will learn a lot about what makes you tick. To be successful many changes may be necessary. The easy ones relate to your attitudes about food and eating. Others involve decisions regarding what is really important in your life; how to prioritize; whether you are willing to take responsibility for the decisions you make and whether you can commit to yourself. To see what I mean, let's listen to what our experts learned about themselves.

Challenges Will Arise, but What Defines You as a Person Is the Way You Respond!

We all know that life is rarely a bowl of cherries. Or, as Erma Bombeck said, "If life is a bowl of cherries, why am I in the pits?" One of her books is titled *The Grass is Always Greener over the Septic Tank*. Despite much adversity in her life, she never took it lying down. Her keen sense of humor and the ability to express it effectively defined her as a person. Putting a positive spin on daily problems, she captured millions of hearts while creating entertainment in the process!

You, too, will encounter many speed bumps during the odyssey on which you are embarking. Make no mistake, there will be difficult times when you feel like throwing in the towel. After a sleepless night you may awaken and trudge to the scale only to find that the needle has not budged in two days; remember a conference call that was not in your Day-Timer; and on your way out the door notice a spot on the carpet that Fido just deposited! A typical day in the life! After cleaning up your doggie's "present," you may be amused that you are still leaving home with a smile on your face. The ability to get beyond what are really short-term hassles must be part of your repertoire.

The Definition of Insanity...

...is doing the same thing over and over again and expecting different results. You have probably heard this saying in many other settings, but it is no less pertinent when you are trying to lose weight, possibly even more so. Diedre S said this epiphany literally changed her life. When she gained weight in the past she had always managed to take it off. Her prior approach had been to eat and drink whatever struck her fancy, gain weight over a three- or four-month period, then starve herself to lose it again.

Lately, after losing interest in this way of dieting, she had put weight on and hadn't been able to take it off. After multiple conversations with her best friend she decided to become more informed about healthy eating habits and to revamp her dietary approach. As a result she feels better, eats in a healthier manner, has lost weight and has even been weaned off several blood pressure and cholesterol lowering medicines. What makes her happiest is that now she isn't confronted with repeated periods of near fasting to lose those unwanted pounds. She had come to dread those days and weeks of feeling hungry all the time and doesn't miss them at all.

The revelation for Michelle R came in a completely different manner. When she enrolled in the clinical trial she was required to attend group sessions that covered an array of topics including exercise options, how to make sensible food choices and what processed foods were and why it was important to limit them in her diet. These all seemed logical. However, she wasn't inclined to waste time on other topics that appeared to be just common sense.

You will encounter many speed bumps during the odyssey on which you are embarking. Make no mistake, there will be difficult times when you feel like throwing in the towel.

One that really surprised her was a discussion about what it meant to feel hungry. Having never thought about it much before, she soon realized that her prior notion of it being caused by an empty stomach wasn't very useful and might have even contributed to her tendency to put on weight.

During this specific meeting there seemed to be as many interpretations as there were participants. What she learned from the spirited conversation that ensued helped her discern in a more subtle fashion a variety of perceptions she had not really appreciated—revelations that made her more aware of the changes her body would soon be experiencing. She realized that what she had previously dreaded actually turned out to be lively and informative sessions filled with pertinent information.

With the exception of having to buy a small scale to measure the weight of a piece of meat or fish and having to use measuring cups to dish out precisely two thirds of a cup of carrots, a quarter cup of almonds or some other quantity of food, Shelly N readily endorsed each of the recommendations. Her initial response had been that these extra steps were a colossal waste of time. Her daily schedule was already over-booked, and she literally found herself arriving late wherever she went. So it made no sense to her to unnecessarily complicate life further.

That is, until she had to estimate an array of portion sizes in front of the other study participants. She soon found that her ability to "guesstimate" what comprised a half-cup or a quarter-pound was far from accurate. Not only was she frequently but she always *underestimated*, so her daily calorie intake about 600 to 800 calories more than she thought—a yet very common finding among most of the study subjects simple demonstration made her a true believer in the use the food scale especially once she learned that it required two hours of hard exercise to burn off all those extra calories hadn't realized she was consuming. After using the measuring devices for four more weeks, Shelly realized she could make more accurate estimates of her portion sizes.

This insight accelerated her weight loss. The renewed success made her even more motivated to stick with the program. And she was not the only one to witness the power of such a simple intervention. What she found quite fascinating was the fact that not only had she been eating 25 percent more calories than she had thought, but despite eating less (after beginning to use her scale and measuring cups) she was not any hungrier.

Self-Esteem Is Key— Don't Let Your Weight Define You as a Person!

A number of the study volunteers had issues regarding self-esteem. As a result many of them shared the misguided belief that "I am not thin enough — I will not good enough." Ostensibly this makes no sense. Yet it is ingrained in our culture. Consider how models, actresses and other females in various ads are depicted. Whether they are advertising cars, cosmetics, beer or cell phones, it seems that thinner is better. Because we live in an age during which this type of information dominates TV, movies, magazines and the Internet, we are all exposed both consciously and subconsciously to the association of a waif-like body with success, beauty and power.

With this type of upbringing and subliminal messaging, it is not surprising that young girls (and boys as well) develop problems of self-esteem as they mature. As time goes by additional life stressors such as financial, work, health and family-related issues may cause body image and one's reaction to it to become increasingly difficult to contend with.

Maddie W was so troubled by *how she reacted to her weight gain* that she was prescribed an antidepressant. Incidentally, among their many other side effects antidepressants can be associated with weight gain and, like all medications, should only be taken under a doctor's care. In Maddie's situation her medication made it more difficult for her to lose weight. This contributed to losing her sense of self-worth and the downward spiral that ensued. Once this type of thing happens, reversing the process can be extremely difficult.

The good news for Maddie was that she had a great sense of humor and even did some stand-up comedy. That provided her with a sounding board for her emotions and allowed her to vent about her life, her situation and how it made her feel. Luckily, at one of her shows she met a wonderfully supportive young man who convinced her that she was indeed a good person. This sincere gesture of support and honesty allowed her to start feeling much better about herself and what she could contribute to society. Once she realized that there was so much more to life than having a stick figure, she started feeling better about herself and became much more successful at meeting her weight loss goals.

Determine What Is Important in Your Life

Concerns about her weight had plagued June D for a long time. Her friends were "on her case," and she was in a tizzy about what to do. She was finding it increasingly difficult to walk the eighteen holes of golf she played every Saturday without feeling somewhat winded. Bending over to do the yard work she loved so dearly was now a chore as well. Her knees had begun popping and had started aching over the past six months. Though she was only fifty years old, it seemed to her that her body was starting to give out. Working in a bank where she spent most of the time at a desk didn't help the situation.

Being a "professional" woman was all she ever wanted. And she was good at what she did. Whenever a problem arose, she was the "go-to girl" for a creative solution. Worried that she was even losing that talent, she started feeling overwhelmed. It seemed like a number of factors had coalesced to make her feel inept, inadequate and intimidated. This was uncharted territory. People had always looked up to her and respected her opinion. She felt like she was losing control.

About that time she went to visit her daughter Randi, who sensed something was awry. After several attempts June finally opened up and the two spoke frankly for a few hours. Randi suggested delegating some work to subordinates (June was a bit of a control freak, which may have been a contributing factor) and taking a "mental health" break to devote time to her personal well-being.

Following Randi's sage advice, she and her husband went to a quiet mountain retreat they had visited frequently during their younger years. Without intrusions from cell phones and business they formulated a plan together. Now that her children were adults June decided to spend time paying attention to her own needs.

She carved out periods during the week that were designated as "private time," which she used to address three issues. The first involved creating some distance between her private life and her professional life. This was particularly difficult because she anticipated it would make her boss think she was slacking off. Interestingly, he supported the change, telling her that for some time he had been hoping she would do something like this. He feared she was a candidate for burnout and thought more balance was needed in her life.

Second, June dearly missed the music that had been a large part of her life when her kids were in school. So, she decided to learn to play the piano because she now had time to dedicate to lessons.

The third thing she wanted to address was her weight. She and several of her friends joined a local gym that offered nutrition classes, free athletic training and even provided ballroom dancing instruction. It was here that she learned about the weight loss study and decided to participate in the trial. Thanks in part to the support of the other study subjects, she soon found herself engaged with a rekindled zest that had been her hallmark prior to her current difficulties. Shortly thereafter she began losing weight and feeling good about things again.

Set Yourself Up for Success!

Although this tip should be self-evident, it is one that is rarely considered when making significant life changes. During one of the weekly group sessions held in conjunction with the weight loss study, it became the subject of some lively discussion. There were seven women and one man in attendance that evening. Samuel J, or Sammy J as he was called, provided the male perspective. He had been in the army for eight years and had never previously had a weight problem. However, now that his activity level had dropped and he was not routinely going on survival weekends, he realized that his pants had gotten tight and he was no longer comfortable tucking his shirts in.

This realization prompted a wardrobe change that included purchasing a group of what he referred to as his "Aloha" shirts. They were basically oversized, floral Hawaiian prints that were worn loosely over pants or shorts. His other investment was his "fat pants." These unique creations have the ability to expand as one's waistline expands. They easily perform this feat thanks to their hidden elastic bands. They were probably designed for both expanding and receding tummies, but in his case were only required for the former.

While in the army, Sammy J was called upon for his logistical prowess. He was the guy who could single-handedly orchestrate mass movements of supplies and personnel. However, such had not always been the case. As a young man he frequently forgot important items, lost things and usually "didn't get it quite right!"

After he joined the military this all changed in a hurry. He was in a platoon that prided itself on "punctuality and perfection." One purchase he made that facilitated this transformation was a computer, which accompanied him everywhere he went. He soon became the master of spreadsheets and documentation. Each and every shoe, pot, pan, bullet and jacket had a number that was entered into his database.

He was told where the items had to be and when they needed to arrive. With this knowledge he coordinated the entire process on his laptop. Using his newfound organizational skills, he increased his productivity dramatically. In doing so, he had set himself up for success. Now he never lost or forgot anything.

This story made Sammy J the envy of the group. It also motivated "his women" in the group to reevaluate their circumstances and identify risk factors that might contribute to dietary failure. After some lively discourse many ideas emerged. Sylvia T said she had a pantry and a freezer full of diet-breaking foods. She was the type of person who had trouble throwing things away and knew many of these foods had outlived their shelf life. As a result, she cleaned house and got rid of them all. Once this was done she went to the store and replenished her larder with healthy foods and snacks such as nuts, seeds, beef jerky and dried fruits. She soon discovered that she was not the only person who had scores of old calorie-dense, nutrient-poor foods stashed around the house. During the discussion it became clear that although such snacks taste good, they do little to suppress appetite and should not be kept as sources of temptation.

Doris C contributed another "weight loss buster." After her husband's sudden death she filled her time watching a series of TV soap operas that started at 11:30 in the morning and continued until dinnertime. While sitting and watching TV all afternoon, she snacked and was not very active. Not only was this bad news for her weight, but she noticed that she was becoming mentally sluggish as well.

Since she and Sylvia lived two blocks from each other, they made a pact to get out and walk together for 45 minutes each day. Because they grew to be quite good friends, their walking regimen continued throughout the winter. Each of them looked forward to the lively conversations that caused the time and the miles to fly by. Both attribute their success to the outdoor activity they shared four or five times a week. Kudos to them for setting themselves up for success!

To Be Successful at Anything (Especially Losing Weight), You Must Be Willing to Make a Commitment to Yourself

Just waking up one morning and saying, "I'm planning to lose 50 pounds and I'm starting today" is not going to be very effective for most people. That is usually an impulsive spur of the moment type of action. When reconsidered later in the day, this type of gesture rarely makes sense for a number of reasons. First of all, it has not been thoroughly thought out and planned. However, in this scenario at least a weight loss goal was stated—50 pounds. That alone is good. But it doesn't sound as if consideration has been given as to how long it will take to accomplish; what changes will need to be made; how they might impact daily schedules and family members; and many other important components of a successful approach. The decision requires a lot more planning before you can effectively commit to it!

Making this type of pact with yourself is sort of like getting married. You must first find out if the two of you are compatible; what you want to accomplish by getting married; whether or not you want children; if so, how many; whether you can afford your goals; how you will divide the obligations and so forth. Only then will you be ready to commit.

Try exercising with a friend!

Usually a marriage is a public ceremony attended by your nearest and dearest friends and family. You are making a proclamation for all to witness. Part of the reason for doing this is for them to share in the joyous event. The other often implicit reason is that life and marriage, like losing weight, take hard work that requires patience, sacrifice and (at times) quite a bit of support.

The agreement you make with yourself to lose weight should be perceived in much the same way. It must be well designed, formulated for success, announced publicly (at least to a few family members and friends) and then endorsed wholeheartedly *by you!* After all, being successful is important and you are worth it!

Spending the time to develop a carefully crafted game plan and making the appropriate arrangements will markedly increase the chances for success. By announcing you are setting a certain goal and intend to attain it within a specified time frame, your friends become part of the plan and will support you. They don't want to fail, nor do they want you to. This type of approach can be a terrific motivator.

After you make a contract with yourself, you must become accountable. Remember, the buck stops on your desk! You are the ultimate decision maker. So, once the rules are outlined, you *must* stick with them. Otherwise there is little point in going through the exercise.

Get in Touch with Your Body

This means different things to different people, but *it is probably the most significant principle that those who stay thin have mastered.* When you begin a new way of eating, what is most important is *becoming aware of the vague, often unfamiliar signals your body will be generating; understanding what they are telling you; and knowing how to respond appropriately.* If you want to be successful at losing weight, getting in touch with your body is essential!

A different activity profile, novel dietary recommendations and alternative nutritional guidelines will combine to produce quite substantial metabolic alterations. Some may occur immediately while others will become apparent only after several weeks. Your body may require some time to adapt to them. It is important to take a moment to understand what these are and how they can influence the way you feel and react. Heightened awareness will facilitate the entire process. Knowing what to look for makes it easier to discern subtle changes at an earlier stage and to avoid misinterpreting them.

To get started let's talk about several of the pathways that will be affected. For any weight loss program to be successful, you must burn more fat than you store. When you gain weight, you are doing just the opposite—storing more fat than you are burning. To reverse this process, you must change the way your body works.

Preventing the development of sticky fat cells is an example of one of these changes. Knowing how to avoid feeling hungry is another. No one is going to stick to any diet if they feel like they are starving all the time. As we have seen, to lose weight without being hungry requires successfully making the transition from using external calories (meaning the food we eat) to internal calories (the fat stored in our pantries). Once this occurs we're home free because many of us have enough fat to last for a very long time.

The best way to achieve this goal is to avoid brain starvation. The brain is a real energy hog—24 hours a day, seven days a week. When it receives sufficient energy, it functions properly and

If you want to be successful at losing weight, getting in touch with your body is essential!

doesn't get hungry. It isn't picky about where the energy comes from, just that there is never a shortage.

Dietary researchers have known for many years that the most potent hunger trigger is a falling blood sugar level. The faster the fall and the greater the descent, the hungrier you'll feel. Since blood sugar levels fluctuate throughout the day, at some times they are high and other times they are low. It's the *transition periods* that are the most important—especially when sugar levels are falling.

As we saw when comparing Jane's breakfast with John's, her sugar levels fell farther and faster than his, so she got hungry sooner than he did. We all require energy to fuel our bodies and prevent fatigue. The problem with using sugary foods to produce this energy is that they are rapidly metabolized with the unwanted downside of making us hungry again a short time later.

Why does this happen? *It is because the body can't differentiate a falling sugar level that is caused by a spike in insulin from that produced by an impending food shortage.* Under either condition the brain panics because it requires an uninterrupted supply of energy and it can't store sugar. Thus, a falling sugar level signals an emergency—an impending energy shortage—and the brain reacts by stimulating the appetite centers under either condition, because it can't tell the difference.

Since blood sugar levels fluctuate throughout the day, at some times they are high and other times they are low. It's the transition periods that are the most important—especially when sugar levels fall.

The best way to stave off hunger is to be able to tap into the energy stored in our pantries. When this is achieved successfully, we make the transition from burning carbs to burning fat and don't get hungry. If not, we head back to the kitchen.

Since the first step in both scenarios is a falling sugar level, similar metabolic signals are generated. For this reason what it feels like when you are *starting* to make the transition to burning fat can resemble the early stages of hunger. In one instance energy levels continue to fall and we start eating again (BAD), while in the other fat comes to the rescue and we use it as a fuel source (GOOD).

Without fully understanding what is happening at this critical time, it is easy to misinterpret the sensation generated by the change from glucose to fat as the preferred fuel source from the feeling of true hunger. This is important because if weight loss is to be achieved, we must not misconstrue how this critical transition feels (and what it means) because we need to be making it with regularity.

The most efficient ways to facilitate this transition are to choose foods that contain slow-release carb sources and to add brain-healthy fats to each meal. The slow-release carbs blunt the fall in sugar while the brain-healthy fats speed up fat burning.

You now know how to properly begin to differentiate feelings of hunger from the changes associated with the transition to fat burning. As you become more attuned to your body, you will more easily be able to sense this vital difference!

Prior bad eating habits have caused us to grow accustomed to interpreting that feeling as hunger because we didn't know how to reliably transition to the other (preferable) energy source—fat. When we begin eating properly and learn how to interpret the metabolic signals being produced, we'll eat less, feel better and lose weight.

The reasons for going into this level of detail regarding the hormonal and metabolic effects of food and how they impact weight gain are central to understanding the basis for the way you will feel. Hopefully, this knowledge will assist you in achieving your weight loss goal.

On a brain-friendly (meaning one that prevents brain starvation)—and waist-friendly—diet, the transitions from one fuel to another are small and appetite is suppressed. However, a subtle transition still occurs. For this reason it is important to remember that such a diet can produce feelings that may be *misinterpreted* as early signs of hunger. However, they are *not* signs of starvation or lack of food, but merely reflect *a transition in the fuel mixture from carbohydrate to fat.*

This is why being in touch with your body, that is, knowing how to interpret what you are feeling, is critical, because *it helps differentiate between a normal metabolic transition and true hunger.* Probably the most meaningful way to describe this subtle distinction in perception is the difference between *wanting* to eat and *needing* to eat. When this difference is appreciated, it is possible to identify the physiological shift from the fat storing to the fat burning state—the condition associated with weight loss!

Nicole R summed it up nicely when she said, "I never felt hungry, because there was *no need* to be hungry!"

Work at It, but Don't Get Depressed

For a number of reasons, becoming a Big Loser is not an easy accomplishment. You must realize there are numerous ways to get to the finish line, many of which are not direct, predictable or easy. Just when things are looking good, you might let up and even gain one or two pounds. This has happened to each of our experts, often more than once! Instead of fearing it, it is best to assume it will happen and learn to deal with it. Part of successfully confronting a wrinkle in your plans is having the mental toughness to work through it. This is where your focus should be. The consensus of the group was that if you approach things this way, you won't get depressed or feel overwhelmed.

The Little Things Can Add Up

Gaining weight is a process that takes a long time, usually measured in years, not months. Conversely, losing a substantial amount of weight takes time, too. Consider the result of gaining a mere five grams of fat each day. That is only 45 calories—about the number in half an apple. However, if that gain is repeated day after day the grams add up. After one year they total almost five pounds. After ten years they add up to fifty pounds, and after twenty years you will find yourself 100 pounds heavier!

By paying attention to the same "little" details, the reverse can also occur. The choice is up to you. The best approach is not one that includes draconian measures, severe caloric restriction or feelings of deprivation. It involves finding a program that makes sense for you and can easily be adhered to and incorporated into your daily schedule. This is the best way to be happy, feel great and lose weight!

10
Weight Loss Gems

You have just heard about the mental approach the weight loss experts in the study found to be most helpful. Now I will pass on some practical suggestions that worked best for them.

Use a Log Book

Each participant in the study was provided with a spiral notebook that was small enough to be easily portable, but large enough to record daily observations including food consumption, activities, stressors, sleep duration and quality, frustrations, questions and suggestions. Dietary choices and activity levels are pillars of any weight loss program and they were recorded assiduously. This diary was referred to as their Log Book and was usually carried around in a purse, knapsack or briefcase. It never left the side of the study volunteer. This was vital for success. When they initially enrolled in the study, many of the volunteers thought keeping a detailed record was a useless inconvenience. However, as the trial progressed this perception changed dramatically. By the end they were all vocal supporters who praised the critical role the Log Books contributed to the success of the weight loss process.

The Biggest Losers each utilized their Log Books differently. However, they all recorded the key items we have been referring to. On a daily basis they measured and recorded the weights and amounts of literally everything they put in their mouths. A typical entry might be:

Salmon—4 ounces

Asparagus stalks—6 with 1 pat of butter

Garden salad—1½ cups

Oil and vinegar dressing with Italian seasoning—2 tsp.

Salt and pepper

Non-sweetened iced tea with 1 slice of lemon (12 ounces)

This level of detail is important if you need to estimate the number of calories consumed or the fat-to-carb ratio.

The Log Book was also used to keep track of all activities. The subjects each wore pedometers that tallied the number of steps they took each day as they went for a walk, did chores around the house, ran up and down the stairs or prepared meals. A similar approach was used for the resistance or weight-training portion of the activity regimen.

Prepare Food Beforehand

When you are really hungry is not a good time to be shopping for or preparing food. That is when you are obsessing about what you can eat immediately. Invariably, you are not going to make optimal food choices under that scenario. You are likely to select whatever can be wolfed down without preparation—"fast food" in its original state.

It is best to undertake food preparation when you have sufficient time to plan and prepare high quality snacks and meals and are not ravenously hungry. You can mix and match high nutrient density, low calorie choices in a creative fashion. Make munchies that are easily transported to work or that you can comfortably eat in the car when you are doing errands. Save those that are more appropriately kept in the refrigerator for home-based snacking. That way sugar, refined carbohydrates and trans fats may be minimized and your waistline will thank you.

Donald N swore by this approach. It prevented him from "going off the edge" many times. He found that if he was able

It is best to prepare food when you have sufficient time to plan and prepare high quality snacks and meals.

to eat some small healthy snack and wait for fifteen minutes, he wouldn't get hungry for hours. He now refers to this as his "fifteen minute" rule. It was so effective that many of the Biggest Losers adopted it.

Eat When You Are Hungry and Never Allow Yourself to Get Too Hungry

Many of our experts detailed what they snacked on if they began to feel hungry. The choices were as different as the participants. Sammy J was a true believer in the celery and peanut butter approach. Michelle swore by beef jerky, saying, "It was chewy, tasty and expanded in my stomach." Kat liked carrying around a mixture of almonds and pumpkin seeds with a few dried cranberries thrown in. She explained, "They provided a slightly salty sweetness that I loved. I ate a handful and felt satisfied for hours! They traveled well and stayed fresh for a long time. My coworkers started doing the same thing. Remarkably, it helped several of them lose ten pounds!"

Marti B said, "After you have crossed the line from realizing you need to eat to the real hunger zone, it's very difficult not to overeat once you start. You go from hanging on by your fingertips to an eating free-fall." She went on to say that one thing that really helped was forgoing alcohol. "I must admit that I like a glass or two of wine with dinner. However, I frequently found that when I had something to drink it was harder to moderate what I ate. I guess my inhibitions were diminished when they needed to be even more discriminating. Alcohol also has a lot of calories! So cutting it out of my diet entirely was very helpful for me."

"Another thing that was very important was distinguishing the difference between how it feels to really be hungry from the false sense of hunger that can arise out of boredom—a response that doesn't merit eating. That might be the most important thing I learned during the support group meetings."

Your Pedometer Will Become Your Friend

"When I first saw it, I had no clue how it worked. I couldn't even turn it on. Once I figured out how to use it, I soon realized how inactive I really was. It taught me a lot. When I finally became used to having it on my belt, I quickly learned how many steps I could add during the course of the day," said Maude F.

This was a typical response from the study participants. "I never realized that little box could help me so much." And it did in several ways. Not just by encouraging more steps per day (steps that could be added very easily while one was doing other necessary things without taking much additional time), but also by the curiosity and support it aroused in people who asked about it as they saw it being worn day after day. A number of friends and coworkers even purchased one for themselves.

The fascinating thing that Trudy W noticed was that coworkers would ask "How far have you walked today?" Or when she looked as if she was on her way to the snack machine, they would head her off and tell her she was doing so well losing weight that they didn't want her to take a step in the wrong direction. They actually became ardent supporters and saved her a number of times, reinforcing her will power in the process.

Reading Labels Is Key!!!

"It's amazing what is hidden in foods to make them taste good. Who would have guessed they put high-fructose corn syrup in ketchup?" remarked Todd B. "What does that have to do

You'll be surprised at how many seemingly "nonessential" ingredients you'll find in prepared foods.

with tomatoes?" he was heard asking in the group session during which a number of packaged foods were scrutinized for hidden and unwanted ingredients. Dottie was shocked that "partially hydrogenated sunflower oil is how trans fats appear on food labels! I knew they were bad, and although I checked every label for them, I didn't know that's what they were called in the food business. I guess they do it that way to pull the wool over our eyes."

Most of the experts say they really benefited from the label-reading exercise. Almost uniformly they reported they were stunned by the hidden amount of salt and sugar in the food they brought home from the grocery store. They were surprised at all the seemingly "nonessential" ingredients such as flavoring agents, colors and stabilizers that are in the groceries that filled their shopping carts. Whether you believe artificial sweeteners are safe or not, you need to be aware of where they are lurking so you can make informed decisions about what you put in your mouth.

So, remember, the next time (and every time thereafter) you go shopping, READ THE LABELS!

A *Treat* Rather Than a *Cheat*

We are not on this planet very long. While some of us *eat to live,* most of us also *live to eat.* In real life we must determine how we organize our schedules, decide what to do and choose how and what to eat. There are no food police looking over our shoulders. Nonetheless, we make many good decisions but also some that seem counterintuitive. Despite knowing what we should be eating, we often make different choices that might not appear to make sense. However, that is part of life, and a part that makes life worth living! (The living to eat part.)

Jodie R had this perspective in mind when she remarked to the group, "I am calling this tiramisu a *treat* and not a *cheat*." What she meant by this was that she had built certain "indiscretions" into her eating approach so she didn't feel guilty when they occurred. She knew what she was doing and made up for it by being scrupulous about what she ate both the day before and the day after. By treating herself for being "good," in her mind that dessert was not a cheat because it was planned for ahead of time. Other dietary choices were altered to appropriately incorporate the treat into her meal so (the best part) she didn't end up feeling guilty about what she had done.

You should compile your own weight loss gems. That way when you are queried about how you did it, you can easily pass along what worked for you!

Part 4

How We Know the Brain–Belly Connection Really Works!

11
Clinical Trials 101

In most other books that talk about how to lose weight, the recommendations are made by people who have an opinion about what works. An opinion can be correct, incorrect or somewhere in between. Promoters of many diets merely provide anecdotal evidence that their diet works—evidence based on reports of a few people using the diet (for example, Jane Smith followed this diet for 2 months and lost 40 pounds!).

Why is it crucial for you to know this? Because anecdotal results can be misleading for a number of reasons: you don't know—how well the diet was followed; whether the weight was lost because of the diet or other extraneous factors; what side effects it caused; what the likelihood is that you will lose weight based on how well other persons did; or what other weight-loss efforts they might have been making in addition to following the diet. If you're going to spend the time and effort to learn about and stick to a diet and exercise program, you certainly want it to make scientific sense, to be safe and to provide exactly what is promised. How else can you be sure that your program will deliver?

Clinical Trials

Studies called clinical trials are conducted to test hypotheses. Hypotheses are basically guesstimates of what might be true— that a certain drug can lower blood pressure, for example. Clinical trials are precise tools that investigate treatment plans, drugs or surgical procedures under controlled circumstances in human subjects who volunteer to be participants. When a study is done this way, the results can usually be applied to a broader audience—assuming the extended group closely resembles the participants in the study. (See *Example: Cancer Drug Clinical Trial* on page 150.)

The clinical trial process should be used when any dietary regimen or nutritional supplement formulation is being studied or compared to conventional recommendations. Why isn't this usually done? For one reason conducting clinical trials is tremendously expensive. For another the most conclusive results are usually obtained when the subjects are in a hospital and have their meals prepared for them so that everyone follows exactly the same diet. A third reason is that clinical trials generally must be conducted for a long time, and not many people volunteer for such a program.

Given these constraints, in most weight-loss trials scientists try to do the best they can to gather meaningful information while study participants live at home and do their own shopping and food preparation. That is the approach we used to evaluate both the diet and activity program described in this book as well as the unique nutritional supplement that was tested.

Our Study Design

A *study design* describes in detail each part of a clinical trial—the purpose of the trial, how subjects are chosen, the detailed steps outlining how the trial is to be performed at each step along the way and how the results are to be analyzed.

Purpose

We wanted to do two things: 1) compare one diet and activity program with another (the Feed Your Brain Lose Your Belly diet and activity program was compared with typical diet and activity regimens used by the volunteers in the clinical study), and 2) see how adding the nutritional supplement Vi-texxa™ impacted the weight-loss effect of the Feed Your Brain Lose Your Belly diet and activity program. To answer these questions we needed three groups of subjects to participate in a double-blind, placebo-controlled clinical trial. These groups are referred to as the three *arms* of the study.

Subjects

To solicit volunteers we relied on television advertising. Interested subjects were then contacted via phone to make sure they understood what being in a clinical trial entailed before inviting them to the clinic for further questioning. Those chosen to participate were randomly assigned to one of the three groups (Group 1, Group 2 or Group 3), but not told which group they were in. Not even the researchers found out who was in which group until the trial ended (hence the term *double-blind*). All were treated equally and were given identical-looking capsules to take every day. Some received capsules containing an inactive product (a placebo); others received the supplement being tested—Vi-texxa™. Some were asked to follow a special diet (the Feed Your Brain Lose Your Belly diet), though none of the groups had caloric restrictions.

Performance

What happened after the subjects enrolled in our study were randomized into one of the three groups? All were followed in an identical fashion: their weight, fat mass, lean mass, blood pressure and heart rate were tested every other week and they were questioned about appetite suppression. They were also evaluated for side effects.

Everyone attended meetings during which questions were answered, dietary understanding was refined and compliance was assessed. (Compliance means how strictly each subject followed the study guidelines.)

EXAMPLE: CANCER DRUG CLINICAL TRIAL

In a clinical trial for a hypothetical new cancer drug, CancerNew, one group of participants was treated with the best conventional drug therapy, CancerOld, and another group with CancerNew.

When clinical trials are performed, three things are very important: that the groups being compared are chosen randomly; that they have similar makeup; and that neither the subjects nor the researchers know which subjects are receiving which drug. (If neither the subjects nor the researchers know who is receiving which drug, the study is described as "double-blind." This safeguard helps prevent the researchers from unintentionally influencing the outcome as a result of their personal beliefs and biases.)

In this hypothetical trial that I'm using as an example, the two groups had a similar age range, a similar proportion of males and females and a similar type and stage of cancer (This is what "similar makeup" in the paragraph above means.). A computer program randomly assigned people to one of the two groups. Although one group was treated with CancerOld and the other with CancerNew, the drugs were formulated to have an identical appearance and neither the subjects nor the researchers knew which drug any of the participants was receiving until the clinical trial had been completed.

After the drugs were given for the prescribed length of time both groups of subjects were evaluated for five years to document recurrence of cancer. Even during this time, neither subjects nor researchers knew who had received CancerNew or CancerOld.

Once the trial was over and the code was broken so that everyone knew which subjects were given each treatment, it was found in those who had received CancerOld that cancer reappeared (on average) after 17 months, while for those who received CancerNew it reappeared after 22 months. Based on these findings, researchers were able to conclude that CancerNew delayed recurrence of this type and stage of cancer, on average, by five months compared to CancerOld the drug that was conventionally being used. Based on these findings, it would be predicted that other people with similar stages of cancer can expect the same types of beneficial results.

At the end of the six week study period final body measurements were taken so that they could be compared to the measurements taken at the beginning of the study (*baseline* measurements).

As is common in clinical trials, this study had what is called a *rolling admission program*, which means that not everyone started the study simultaneously. Every week four or five subjects volunteered, were screened and were enrolled in the study. So, once the initial group of subjects had finished, four or five additional participants completed the trial every week.

Analysis

After each volunteer completed the study program, all of the information that was collected during the clinical trial was entered into a computer program that analyzed the changes in the study parameters we were evaluating—such things as weight loss, fat loss, assessment of appetite suppression and so forth. Then the results were compiled and tabulated.

Next, the effect of the Feed Your Brain Lose Your Belly diet and activity program, both alone and when used in conjunction with the nutritional supplement Vi-texxa™, were evaluated.

Each of the three groups was large enough so that when the code was broken at the end of the trial we could determine with a high level of certainty, using sophisticated statistical analysis, whether one group performed better than another with regard to weight and fat loss, appetite changes, etc.

Description of the Feed Your Brain Lose Your Belly Groups

Group 1: Those enrolled in Group 1 ate what they felt was a healthy diet throughout the study and followed their own activity regimen, which involved approximately the same level of exertion

> ### CLINICAL TRIAL TERMS YOU SHOULD KNOW
>
> The study design we used is called a **prospective, double-blind, randomized, placebo-controlled human clinical trial** - quite a mouthful!
>
> **Prospective** means the study is going forward in time. Subjects are chosen specifically to fit the study description and must follow the study regimen. (**Retrospective** studies examine documentation that has been created in the past (i.e., looking at information that has already been gathered), before study descriptions have been written.)
>
> **Double-blind** means that neither the participants nor the study coordinators (staff conducting the study) know who is receiving placebo or active product. This helps maintain objectivity throughout the trial for everyone—i.e., all the subjects and the researchers, too.
>
> **Randomized** refers to the fact that subjects are not preferentially placed in any specific group. They are randomly assigned to their respective group by a computer program.
>
> **Placebo-controlled** means that the active medication or nutritional supplement looks identical to the inactive product (the placebo), and no one knows which is which (placebo or active product).
>
> This **prospective, double-blind, randomized, placebo-controlled** approach is referred to as the "gold standard" of scientific research. It is more believable than other types of proof when determining whether a product or process works. That is why so much time and effort went into the design and implementation of our study protocol.

as in those of the other two groups. They received placebo (inactive) capsules (although they didn't know it until after the trial).

Group 2: Those in Group 2 also received placebo capsules that contained no active ingredients to promote weight loss. In addition they were asked to follow a particular diet and exercise program (the Feed Your Brain Lose Your Belly diet and activity program that included walking with a pedometer for about 30 to 50 minutes three times a week, doing 20 minutes of light resistance training for two days each week and doing a few minutes of balance training each week).

Group 3: Those in Group 3 followed the same diet and exercise regimen as did the subjects in Group 2. The only difference between the two groups was that those subjects in Group 3 received the product Vi-texxa™ instead of a placebo.

Again, no one in any of the groups and no one administering the clinical trial knew which capsules (placebo or Vi-texxa™) any of the subjects were receiving while the study was in progress.

You can see that the only difference between Group 2 and Group 3 was that Group 2 took the placebo and Group 3 took Vi-texxa™. Both Group 2 and Group 3 followed the same Feed Your Brain Lose Your Belly diet and activity program.

Group 1 ate and exercised as they usually did and took a placebo capsule. Thus, the only difference between Group 1 and Group 2 was their diet and exercise regimen because they both took the placebo product (although during the study the participants didn't know what they were taking).

The difference between Group 1 and Group 3 was that Group 3 used the Food Your Brain Lose Your Belly diet and activity program and took Vi-texxa™ instead of following the conventional diet and exercise program and taking placebo—as Group 1 did. Therefore, any differences in outcome between Groups 1 and 3 must be attributed to the combined effects of the Feed Your Brain Lose Your Belly diet/activity program and the nutritional supplement Vi-texxa™. Differences in outcome between Groups 2 and 3 could be attributed only to the fact that Group 3 subjects took Vi-texxa™ rather than the placebo product, which Group 2 was given.

The Code Is Broken!

After all participants had completed each phase of the study, the clinical investigators entered all of the data into a large database that included baseline weight, weight measurements taken every other week, baseline fat mass, fat mass taken every other week, blood pressure, heart rate, assessment of appetite, compliance, answers from questionnaires and evaluations to determine whether there were any adverse effects from the supplement formulation. A host of baseline demographic and medical information including age, height, smoking history, presence of existing medical conditions, and so forth was also input in the database. Comparisons between each subject's baseline values and values at the end of the study were then computed.

Finally, after all of the data were entered the study code was broken so that researchers could find out who was in each of the three arms of the clinical trial and determine whether there were any significant differences in their outcomes. Averages for each group were calculated and compared.

[Note: The details of this type of analysis can tax the brains of even the most mathematically gifted. Here we will present only the results of that analysis.]

The Results of the Feed Your Brain Lose Your Belly Diet and Activity Program

In this section we will examine the results attributable to the Feed Your Brain Lose Your Belly diet and activity program and will not be evaluating the effect of the weight loss supplement Vi-texxa™. That will be discussed in the next section.

During the six-week trial period subjects in Group 1 remained essentially weight-stable, losing on average 0.04 pounds (less than an ounce) in six weeks.

Those on the Feed Your Brain Lose Your Belly diet and activity program lost, on average, 4.4 pounds in six weeks. This means the Feed Your Brain Lose Your Belly diet and activity program alone was responsible for an average weight loss of 4.36 (4.40 – 0.04) pounds over six weeks compared to the conventional diet followed by those subjects in Group 1. That amounts to 0.73 pounds (almost three-quarters of a pound) per week! These results were *statistically significant* (meaning that according to scientific standards, they are unlikely to have happened due to chance).

More importantly, calculations for fat loss over the six-week trial showed that the Group 1 subjects *gained* 0.35 pounds of fat while the Group 2 subjects lost an average of 4.30 pounds of fat. Thus, persons in Group 2 each lost an average of 4.65 (4.30 + 0.35) pounds of fat in six weeks compared to the Group 1 subjects—an average of 0.77 pounds of fat loss per week.

The researchers also looked at the *percentage* of subjects in each group who lost more than five pounds of weight during the study and found that only 6 percent of the Group 1 subjects accomplished this, while 40 percent of the Group 2 subjects did.

Figure 11.1: Weight Loss for Conventional vs. Feed Your Brain, Lose Your Belly

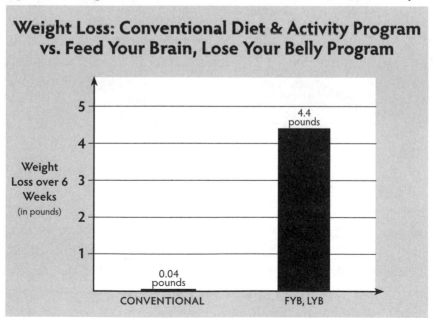

What You Should Know

The take-home message is that the Feed Your Brain LoseYour Belly diet and activity program was responsible for almost five pounds (4.65 pounds to be exact) of fat loss over the 6-week course of the study.

The Results of the Nutritional Product Vi-texxa™

You saw above how successful the Feed Your Brain Lose Your Belly diet and activity program (when used alone) was at producing weight and fat loss. In this section we will discuss differences between the outcomes of Groups 1 and 3 and between Groups 2 and 3.

Group 2 vs. Group 3: The only difference between these groups is that the subjects in Group 3 were given Vi-texxa™, so any differences in outcome between these groups are attributable to the nutritional product.

As we saw previously, the subjects in Group 2 lost an average of 4.40 pounds over six weeks. The average weight loss for group 3 was 11.77 pounds over six weeks—7.37 pounds more than Group 2—an average of an *additional* 1.23 pounds of weight loss per week. This weight loss can be attributed solely to the effects of Vi-texxa™ because Groups 2 and 3 were on the same diet and activity program.

As you probably know, some diets have a greater effect on water weight loss than fat loss. If you've ever yo-yo dieted, I suspect you noticed how quickly your weight jumped back up if your loss was primarily water weight. So, your goal is likely to be to lose as much fat as possible. With that in mind, let's compare fat loss between the two groups. Group 2 subjects lost an average of 4.3 pounds of fat. Group 3 subjects lost 10.42 pounds of fat. This 6.12-pound difference (1.02 pounds per week difference) is attributable to Vi-texxa™ alone and demonstrates that 83 percent of the weight loss due to Vi-texxa™ was fat loss, not water loss.

It should also be noted that *all* the subjects in Group 3 lost weight during the trial! It is rare for all of the participants in any weight loss trial to lose weight—generally some of the volunteers remain stable or even gain weight during a study. These findings suggest, but do not prove, that most persons who follow the Feed Your Brain Lose Your Belly diet and activity program while taking Vi-texxa™ will lose weight.

Figure 11.2: Appetite Suppression with and without Vi-texxa™

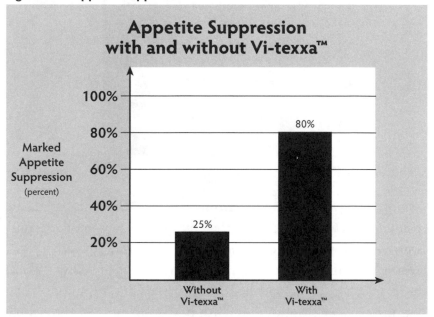

All study subjects were asked about appetite suppression. By comparing the appetite suppression in Groups 2 and 3, we can determine how powerful an appetite suppressant Vi-texxa™ is. Twenty-five percent of those enrolled in Group 2 had marked appetite suppression, as compared to an astounding 80 percent of those in Group 3. This difference is statistically significant and is obviously of great importance for weight loss. Clearly, eating and food consumption increase caloric intake, so anything that decreases appetite should help curtail food consumption and speed weight loss.

Figure 11.3: Weight Loss: Control Diet vs. Feed Your Brain + Vi-texxa™

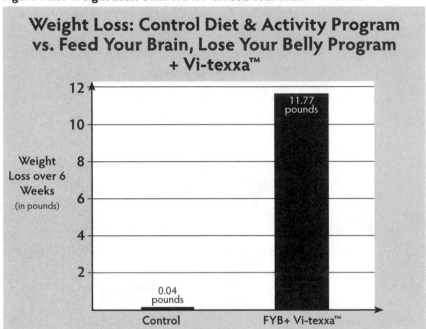

Group 1 vs. Group 3: When Groups 1 and 3 are compared, the results reflect the benefits of the combination of the Feed Your Brain Lose Your Belly diet and activity program and Vi-texxa™. Group 3 lost an average of 11.73 pounds (1.95 pounds per week) more than Group 1, and had a fat loss of 10.77 pounds (1.80 pounds per week) more than Group 1. And most of the people in Group 3 also reported a marked reduction in appetite. It is also apparent from the analysis that 92 percent of the weight loss was actually fat loss, not water loss!

Table 11.1: Summary of Clinical Trial Results

GROUP	WEIGHT LOSS (LBS)	APPETITE SUPPRESSION (%)
1	0.04	0
2	4.40	25
3	11.77	80

The Bottom Line

The bottom line is that in conjunction with Vi-texxa™, the Feed Your Brain Lose Your Belly diet and activity program produced large weight and fat loss and achieved marked appetite suppression! This is good news indeed! It demonstrates how well the Vi-texxa™ nutritional supplement and the Feed Your Brain Lose Your Belly diet and activity program work together.

Now you are armed with the insight of a scientist and are ready to understand how to read and decipher the results of human clinical trials! Knowing how clinical trials are performed will help you not only to accurately interpret results from weight loss studies, but also to evaluate news briefs from magazines, the Internet and newspaper articles. In other words it will help you to see through the fluff, make sense of what is being presented and separate real science from pseudo-science.

• • •

One of the things that keeps scientists honest, so to speak, is publishing the results of their research and clinical trials in peer-reviewed journals. Not all of the articles that are submitted are accepted for publication in these journals. Prior to publication the articles are read by a review committee of unrelated scientists, who may be M.D.s, Ph.D.s or both, to determine whether each article merits publication based on both the quality of content and level of interest in the subject. The results of our clinical trial were published in a peer-reviewed medical journal called *The Internet Journal of Nutrition and Wellness*. The article (written by the person who performed the study, Dr. James Blum) was titled "Evaluation of a Combined Approach to Weight Loss." Although Vi-texxa™ is not mentioned by name, it was the product being studied. To access the article, please go to: http://www.ispub .com/journal/the_internet_journal_of_nutrition_and_wellness/ volume_7_number_1_21/article/evaluation_of_a_combined_ approach_to_weight_loss.html

Suggested Reading

Berry, M. N., D. G. Clark, A. R. Grivell, and P. G. Wallace. "The Contribution of Hepatic Metabolism to Diet-Induced Thermogenesis." *Metabolism* 34 (1985): 141–147.

Biessels, G. J., B. Bravenboer, and W. H. Gispen. "Glucose, Insulin and the Brain: Modulation of Cognition and Synaptic Plasticity in Health and Disease: A Preface." *European Journal of Pharmacology* 490 (2004): 1–4.

Boden, G., K. Sargrad, C. Homko, M. Mozzoli, and T. P. Stein. "Effect of a Low-Carbohydrate Diet on Appetite, Blood Glucose Levels, and Insulin Resistance in Obese Patients with Type 2 Diabetes." *Ann Int Med* 142 (2005): 403–411.

Byrnes, Stephen. "Are Saturated Fats Really Dangerous for You?" http://www.mercola.com/2002/feb/23/vegetarianism_myths_06.htm

Cahill, G. F. Jr, and R. L. Veech. "Ketoacids? Good Medicine?" *Trans Am Clin Climatol Assoc* 114 (2003): 149–161.

Carro, E., and I. Torres-Aleman. "The Role of Insulin and Insulin-like Growth Factor 1 in the Molecular and Cellular Mechanisms Underlying the Pathology of Alzheimer's Disease." *European Journal of Pharmacology* 490 (2004): 127-133.

Convit, A., O. T. Wolf, C. Tarshish, and M. J. de Leon. "Reduced Glucose Tolerance is Associated with Poor Memory Performance and Hippocampal Atrophy Among Normal Elderly." *Proceedings of the National Academy of Sciences of the United States of America* 100 (2003): 2019–2022.

Craft, S. "Insulin Resistance and Cognitive Impairment." *Archives of Neurology* 62 (2005): 1043–1044.

Craft, S. "Insulin Resistance Syndrome and Alzheimer's Disease: Age- and Obesity-Related Effects on Memory, Amyloid and Inflammation." *Neurobiology of Aging* 26S (2005): S65–S69.

Craft, S., and G. S. Watson. "Insulin and Neurodegenerative Disease: Shared and Specific Mechanisms." *Lancet* 3 (2004): 169–178.

Cunnane, S. C. "New Developments in Alpha-Linolenate Metabolism with Emphasis on the Importance of Beta-Oxidation and Carbon Recycling." *World Rev Nutr Diet* 88 (2001): 178–183.

Cunnane, S. C. "Problems with Essential Fatty Acids: Time for a New Paradigm?" *Prog Lipid Res* 42 (2003): 544–568.

Cunnane, S. C. "Metabolic and Health Implications of Moderate Ketosis and the Ketogenic Diet." *Prostaglandins, Leukotrienes and Essential Fatty Acids* 70 (2004): 233–234.

Cunnane, S. C. "Metabolism of Polyunsaturated Fatty Acids and Ketogenesis: An Emerging Connection." *Prostaglandins, Leukotrienes and Essential Fatty Acids* 70 (2004) 237–241.

Enig, Mary. *Know Your Fats: The Complete Primer for Understanding the Nutrition of Fats, Oils and Cholesterol.* Bethesda: Bethesda Press, 2000.

Fishel, M. A., G. S. Watson, T. J. Montine, Q. Wang, P. S. Green, J. J. Kulstad, D. G. Cook, E. R. Peskind, L. D. Baker, D. Goldgaber, W. Nie, S. Asthana, S. R. Plymate, and S. Craft. "Hyperinsulinemia Promotes Synchronous Increases in Central Inflammation and Beta-Amyloid in Normal Adults." *Archives of Neurology* 62 (2005): 1539–1544.

Freemantle, E., M. Vandal, J Tremblay-Mercier, S. Tremblay, J. C. Blachere, M. E. Begin, J. T. Brenna, A. Windust, and S. C. Cunnane. "Omega-3 Fatty Acids, Energy Substrates and Brain Function During Aging." *Prostaglandins, Leukotrienes and Essential Fatty Acids* 75 (2006): 213–220.

Gardner, C. D., A. Kiazand, S. Alhassan, S. Kim, R. S. Stafford, R. R. Balise, H. C. Kraemer, and A. C. King. "Comparison of the Atkins, Zone, Ornish, and LEARN Diets for Change in Weight and Related Risk Factors Among Overweight Premenopausal Women." *JAMA* 297 (2007): 969–977.

Geroldi, C., G. B. Frisoni, G. Paolisso, S. Bandinelli, J. M. Guralnik, and L. Ferrucci. "Insulin Resistance in Cognitive Impairment." *Archives of Neurology* 62 (2005): 1067–1072.

Haist, R. E., and C. H. Best. "Carbohydrate Metabolism and Insulin." In *The Physiological Basis of Medical Practice,* 8th edition. (pp. 1329–1367) Edited by C. H. Best and N. M. Taylor. Baltimore: Williams and Wilkins, 1996.

Han, J. R., B. Deng, J. Sun, C. G. Chen, B. E. Corkey, J. L. Kirkland, J. Ma, and W. Guo. "Effects of Dietary Medium-Chain Triglyceride on Weight Loss and Insulin Sensitivity in a Group of Moderately Overweight Free-Living Type 2 Diabetic Chinese Subjects." *Metabolism* 56 (2007): 985–991.

Hanssen, P. "Treatment of Obesity by a Diet Relatively Poor in Carbohydrates." *Acta Medica Scandinavica* 88 (1936): 97–106.

Henderson, S. T. "High Carbohydrate Diets and Alzheimer's disease." *Medical Hypotheses* 62 (2004): 689–700.

Kahn, B. B., and J. Flier. "Obesity and Insulin Resistance." *J Clin Invest* 106 (2000): 473–481.

Kasai, M., H. Maki, N. Nosaka, T. Aoyama, K. Ooyama, H. Uto, M. Okazaki, O. Igarashi, and K. Kondo. "Effect of Medium-Chain Triglycerides on the Postprandial Triglyceride Concentration in Healthy Men." *Biosci Biotechnol Biochem* 67 (2003): 46–53.

Keys, A., J. Brozek, A. Henschel, O. Mickelsen, and H. L. Taylor. *The Biology of Human Starvation.* 2 vols. Minneapolis: University of Minnesota Press, 1950.

McCall, A. L. "Altered Glycemia and Brain-Uptake and Potential Relevance to the Aging Brain." *Neurobiology of Aging* 26S (2005): S70–S75.

McGarry, J. D., and D. W. Foster. "Regulation of Hepatic Fatty Acid Oxidation and Ketone Body Production." *Annu Rev Biochem* 49 (1980): 395–420.

Mokdad, A. H., B. A. Bowman, E. S. Ford, F. Vinicor, J. S. Marks, and J. P. Koplan. "The Continuing Epidemic of Obesity in the United States." *JAMA* 284 (2000): 1650–1651.

Mokdad, A. H., M. K. Serdula, W. H. Dietz, B. A. Bowman, J. S. Marks, and J. P. Koplan. "The Spread of the Obesity Epidemic in the United States, 1991-1998." *JAMA* 282 (1999): 1519–1522.

Morris, M. C., D. A. Evans, J. L. Bienias, C. C. Tangney, D. A. Bennett, R. S. Wilson, N. Aggarwal, and J. Schneider. "Consumption of Fish and N-3 Fatty Acids and Risk of Incident Alzheimer Disease." *Archives of Neurology* 60 (2003): 940–946.

Morris, M. C., D. A. Evans, C. C. Tangney, J. L. Bienias, and R. S. Wilson. "Fish Consumption and Cognitive Decline with Age in a Large Community Study." *Archives of Neurology* 62 (2005): 1849–1853.

Reaven, G. M. "The Insulin Resistance Syndrome: Definition and Dietary Approaches to Treatment." *Annual Review of Nutrition* 25 (2005): 391–406.

Reaven, G. A. "Banting Lecture1988: Role of Insulin Resistance in Human Disease." *Diabetes* 37 (1988): 1595–1607.

Reger, M. A., S. T. Henderson, C. Hale, B. Cholerton, L. D. Baker, G. S. Watson, K. Hyde, D. Chapman, and S. Craft. "Effects of Beta-Hydroxybutyrate on Cognition in Memory-Impaired Adults." *Neurobiology of Aging* 25 (2004): 311–314.

Reger, M. A., G. S. Watson, W. H. Frey, L. D. Baker, B. Cholerton, M. L. Keeling, D. A. Belongia, M. A. Fishel, S. R. Plymate, G. D. Schellenberg, M. M. Cherrier, and S. Craft. "Effects of Intranasal Insulin on Cognition in memory-Impaired Older Adults: Modulation by APOE Genotype." *Neurobiology of Aging* 27 (2006) 451–458.

Ruderman, N., D. Chisholm, X. Pi-Sunyer, and S. Schneider. "The "Metabolically-Obese, Normal-Weight Individual Revisited." *Diabetes* 47 (1998): 699–713.

Ruderman, N. B., S. H. Schneider, and P. Berchtold. "The "Metabolically-Obese, Normal-Weight Individual." *Am J Clin Nutr* 34 (1981): 1617–1622.

Scharrer, E. "Control of Food Intake by Fatty Acid Oxidation and Ketogenesis." *Nutrition* 15 (1999): 704–714.

Shishodia, S., G. Sethi, and B. A. Aggarwal. "Curcumin: Getting Back to the Roots." *Annals of the New York Academy of Science* 1056 (2005): 206–217.

St-Onge, M. P., and A. Bosarge. "Weight-Loss Diet that Includes Consumption of Medium-Chain Triacylglycerol Oil Leads to a Greater Rate of Weight and Fat Loss than Does Olive Oil." *Am J Clin Nutr* 87 (2008): 621–626.

St-Onge, M. P., A. Bosarge, L. L. Goree, and B. Darnell. "Medium Chain Triglyceride Oil Consumption as Part of a Weight Loss Diet Does not Lead to an Adverse Metabolic Profile When Compared With Olive Oil." *J Am Coll Nutr* 27 (2008): 547–552.

St-Onge, M. P., R. Ross, W. D. Parsons, and P. J. Jones. "Medium-Chain Triglycerides Increase Energy Expenditure and Decrease Adiposity in Overweight Men." *Obes Res* 11 (2003): 395–402.

Taubes, Gary. *Good Calories, Bad Calories: Challenging the Conventional Wisdom on Diet, Weight Control, and Disease.* New York: Knopf, 2007.

Yehuda, S., S. Rabinovitz, and D. I. Mostofsky. "Essential Fatty Acids and the Brain: From Infancy to Aging." *Neurobiology of Aging* 26, suppl. 1 (2005): 98–102

Yehuda, S. "Omega-6/Omega-3 Ratio and Brain-Related Functions." *World Review of Nutrition and Dietetics* 92 (2003): 37–56.

Veech, R. L. "The Therapeutic Implications of Ketone Bodies: The Effects of Ketone Bodies in Pathological Conditions: Ketogenic Diet, Redox States, Insulin Resistance and Mitochondrial Metabolism." *Prostaglandins, Leukotrienes and Essential Fatty Acids* 70 (2004): 309–319.

Veech, R. L., B. Chance, Y. Kashiwaya, H. A. Lardy, and G. F. Cahill Jr. "Ketone Bodies, Potential Therapeutic Uses." *IUBMB Life* 51 (2001): 241–247.

Appendix

Scientific Research Applied to Dietary Supplements

James M. Blum, Ph.D.

Introduction

This guide is offered to those interested in the field of dietary supplement research and marketing. Reputable individuals involved in the research, production and marketing of dietary supplements take research standards very seriously. First, there is the matter of formulating a supplement blend that is meant to benefit consumers in some way. Second, there is a rigorous and meticulous means of testing the product to determine if it actually has the intended effect. Finally, using published research data, supplement companies develop marketing strategies that promote the real benefit of their product to consumers who purchase it. The following orientation material is provided to aid non-scientific personnel in the understanding of the application of research to promote new products that benefit consumers and to support the reasoned and fact-based marketing of dietary supplements to consumers.

This guide is not meant to instruct lay persons how to conduct research. Only basic information is contained here. All dietary supplement research should be conducted by a credentialed investigator with experience in the type of research being conducted.

The terms *scientist* and *investigator* used in this document refer to the credentialed individual supervising or personally conducting the research study. *Supplement companies* refer to those who offer branded dietary supplements to consumers through sales.

Epidemiology Defined

We find that we cannot improve on the definition of *epidemiology* offered by Wikipedia:

Epidemiology is the study of factors affecting the health and illness of populations, and serves as the foundation and logic of interventions made in the interest of public health and preventive medicine. It is considered a cornerstone methodology of public health research and is highly regarded in evidence-based medicine for identifying risk factors for disease and determining optimal treatment approaches to clinical practice. (Wikipedia 2007)

Scientific Research

Scientific research is the study of scientific matters using what is called the scientific method. According to Merriam Webster's Online Dictionary, the *scientific method* is:

the principles and procedures for the systematic pursuit of knowledge involving the recognition and formulation of a problem, the collection of data through observation and experiment, and the formulation and testing of hypotheses. (Webster's Online Dictionary 2007)

Wikipedia presents a complete and concise expansion of the concept:

Scientific method is a body of techniques for investigating phenomena and acquiring new knowledge, as well as for correcting and integrating previous knowledge. It is based on gathering observable, empirical and measurable evidence subject to specific principles of reasoning, the collection of data through observation and experimentation, and the formulation and testing of hypotheses. Although procedures vary from one field of inquiry to another, identifiable features distinguish scientific inquiry from other methodologies of knowledge. Scientific researchers propose hypotheses as explanations of natural or artificial phenomena and design experimental studies that test these hypotheses for accuracy. These steps must be repeatable in order to predict dependably any future results. Theories that encompass wider domains of inquiry may bind many hypotheses together in a coherent structure. This in turn may assist in the formation of new hypotheses, as well as in placing groups of hypotheses into a broader context of understanding. Among other facets shared by the various fields of inquiry is the conviction that the process must be objective to reduce a biased interpretation of the results. Another basic expectation is to document, archive and share all data and methodology so it is available for careful scrutiny by other scientists, thereby allowing other researchers the opportunity to verify results by attempting to reproduce them. This also allows statistical measures of the reliability of these data to be established. (Wikipedia 2007)

How Scientific Research Applies to Dietary Supplement Trials

Regulation

Federal laws under the purview of the United States Food and Drug Administration (FDA) govern medicine and dietary supplement testing on human subjects in the U.S. All human subject research conducted by universities, hospitals or independent scientists must follow standards that are both comprehensive and complex. One of the many requirements aimed at ensuring safety and unbiased research results is that the study must be approved and overseen by an institutional review board (IRB). These independent boards are formed and commissioned by large medical facilities and universities. All scientific research using human subjects must have the sponsorship of an IRB. Boards vary in size but typically have ten to fifteen members—medical doctors, researchers, nursing professionals, university professors, etc.

A recent development that has greatly eliminated some duplicative administrative expense of numerous local boards is the development of the Central Institutional Review Board (CIRB) Initiative, sponsored by the National Cancer Institute (NCI) in consultation with the Department of Health and Human Services (DHHS) Office for Human Research Protections (OHRP). The CIRB provides an innovative approach to human subject protection through a "facilitated review" process that can streamline local IRB reviews of human subject research. This development eliminates the need for numerous local boards while ensuring study quality and ethics. Individuals who wish to conduct human-subject trials must apply to an appropriate IRB and receive approval to proceed. All professional scientific investigators maintain a relationship with the CIRB or a local IRB in their area.

Human Subject Safety and Ethical Considerations

The principles of scientific research apply to every aspect of dietary supplement testing. From the scientific viewpoint, there is one important principle guiding supplement research to ensure the safe and ethical testing of products using human subjects. Medical research may involve laboratory studies using various materials and tools, animal subjects or human subjects. The study of human subjects has historically been carefully regulated by the scientific community in the United States and around the world. Safeguarding human subjects involves:

- Selecting people who do not have an underlying condition that might be worsened by the research;

- Ensuring that the product has no documented, historical, ill-effects to consumers;

- Ensuring that subjects have the capacity to provide informed consent;

- Ensuring that subjects indicate that consent via a signature; and

- Carefully following the subjects during the course of the trial to ensure their health and safety.

In summary, the study must ensure that the benefit to consumers is commensurate with or reasonable for any risk of negative effect that might result.

Efficacy

The practical goal of supplement testing is to determine whether the supplement actually achieves the intended or claimed results. For example, testing a weight-loss supplement will presumably indicate whether the supplement works in the manner intended; that it can be safely used in certain doses; and that study results are not due to coincidental matters. One characteristic of high-standard research is the use of control subjects. Using this method, a group with similar characteristics is selected and randomly assigned to receive a placebo (inactive look-alike product) or to receive the supplement being tested. This serves to remove the possibility of psychological factors affecting the results because the subjects do not know whether they are getting the placebo or the supplement.

Dietary supplement testing has been viewed with some skepticism by the medical industry and consumers because of a perceived lack of rigorous testing. Reputable supplement-research firms are dedicated to ensuring that the same testing procedures used in medical research are carefully applied to the study of dietary supplement research.

While this type of research requires time and resources, public safety and consumer interests require that supplement companies devote the time and money to quality research of supplements marketed to consumers.

Scientific Research Components

The following terms and phrases make up the common components of scientific research as applied to dietary supplements. They are listed in alphabetical order for ease of reader reference.

Acquisition of Subjects

The acquisition of appropriate subjects is a complex process balancing compliance with FDA regulations, IRB requirements and the financial investment in a supplement that may not yet have gone to market. In addition, the matter of logistics involved in identifying subjects who meet the inclusion and exclusion criteria considering the administrative logistics is a combination of science and art. Acquiring subjects from among friends, employees, acquaintances, friends of employees, or other related scenarios clearly violate FDA guidelines and can put the study in jeopardy. Technically, this can lead to legal action against the owners, physicians associated with the product, marketers, and others associated with the product—it is NOT to be taken lightly.

Some investigators advertise for potential subjects using various media. This can bring study needs to a wide audience in a short period. Using this method, one can note the age and qualifying criteria and ask potential subjects to call for further information. Any method that identifies a random sample of individuals in a particular area may be used.

The process of handling potential subjects is outlined in the research protocol and follows FDA guidelines.

Adverse Events (ADE)

Adverse events are reportable to the IRB and to the company sponsoring the clinical trial. ADEs fall into two major categories: minor and serious. An example of a minor adverse event might be a one- or two-time belching after taking the assigned product. Examples of serious adverse events include gastrointestinal issues, rashes, vertigo, palpitations, abnormal laboratory values and the like. The medical team makes a recommendation that the adverse event be identified as most likely not related to the trial, possibly related, or definitely related to the trial.

A common scenario is that an individual subject may experience a cold or 24-hour flu during the trial. Initially, it may appear to be related but if the symptoms abate quickly (24–36 hours) and do not reappear after additional dosages are consumed, it is generally deemed likely not to be related to the treatment. A rare event may include true cardiac disease such as palpitations or a myocardial infarction ("heart attack"), situations in which the results may be more difficult to categorize. Another less common scenario occurs when a subject receives a diagnosis of a serious illness such as cancer during the trial. Most serious diseases develop over a long period of time and are not due to the supplements under study. Professional investigators have a medical background that allows them to make recommendations to the IRB relative to any ADEs that occur.

Baseline Characteristics

In a study of two or more groups, analyzing the baseline characteristics is the most important method that we can use to determine if the randomization of subjects into the various groups was unbiased or successful. Examples of baseline characteristics may include:

- Age, height, and weight
- Medical conditions such as:
  - Arthritis
  - Asthma
  - Depression
  - Diabetes

– Gastrointestinal conditions

– Heart disease

– Thyroid deficiencies

• Behavioral choices such as alcohol and tobacco use

If the vast majority of these characteristics show a similar distribution pattern between the groups, one concludes that the randomization was adequate and that no obvious bias is present.

The interpretation of these analyses is somewhat delicate since even one or two unequal variables may present a challenge to the interpretation of a study. For example, in a diet or weight management study if the placebo group had an unequal (higher) percentage of those with diabetes and thyroid disease one may be concerned that the placebo group had a more difficult time losing weight independent of the treatment arm to which they were assigned. If on the other hand, the treatment group had higher rates of these conditions and still lost more weight than the placebo group, it would indicate that the product might actually perform better in a larger population sample.

Baseline Testing

Baseline testing refers to the testing of subjects at the beginning of the study to establish a specific baseline measure with which the results or outcomes of the study will be compared. The baseline data are just as important as the final data points and in some cases two sets of baseline data are obtained. This helps to determine whether subjects are too variable to be allowed to continue. For example, in a study based on laboratory values, if two baselines differ by more than 25 percent, the subject may be disqualified from entering the active phase of the study. This step helps ensure a higher chance of detecting a difference if one exists.

Biases

Bias can severely damage supplement research and the credibility of both the product and the company that sells it. It is the job of the qualified, ethical investigator to apply his or her training and expertise to identify and prevent bias from influencing a current study or to uncover overlooked bias that has influenced a past study. In the event of past study review, an investigator is retained to decide if bias has adversely influenced a given study, and if bias is found, to what extent.

Wikipedia defines bias as a "prejudice in the sense for having a preference to one particular point of view or ideological perspective" (Wikipedia 2007). The most common form of bias identified in supplement research is that of a self-fulfilling prophecy in which subjective desire for a certain outcome drives the underlying aspects of the study. Consumers are naturally skeptical of companies that claim their product solves a problem previously thought to be difficult or requiring hard work by simply taking a pill.

One form of research bias is *subject-selection bias* whereby subjects are inappropriately selected for the study. An example would be a diet study that does not exclude subjects with thyroid abnormalities. Since abnormal thyroid function could make losing weight easier or more difficult than for those without the condition, these subjects might bias the study. This type of bias is prevented through careful development of inclusion and exclusion criteria and the consistent application of these criteria.

A *systematic bias* occurs when the study is flawed in its overall procedure, thereby resulting in a study that does not actually measure the desired factors. This is prevented by expert study design and implementation.

Interviewer bias is when an investigator conducts interviews that are influenced by his or her subjective judgments. This is prevented through training and research tools that minimize subjectivity.

Overt professional bias is at play when an unqualified or unscrupulous investigator designs a study biased toward achieving the desired result.

Confounding Variables

In epidemiological terms, a *confounding variable* is a variable that may influence study outcomes but may not have been acknowledged or accounted for in original research. In a study in which it appears that there are positive results due to the product studied, confounding variables can contaminate the study findings because they bring up other potential causes for the positive results (instead of the product that is being tested). Failure to treat confounders carefully or thoroughly may damage the interpretation of a study. An example might be a large national study of cholesterol-lowering drugs. Even if one controls for diet and consistent medication dosing, regional variations in the type and nature of food available in each area may affect the study result. Regional variations in the nature and type of foods available would be a confounding variable.

Being aware of potential confounders allows the investigator to control for them thus making an "apples to apples" comparison possible. In the example of regional food quality, the investigator could isolate regions and study the data within each region.

Potential confounders are identified and accounted for in advance, as much as possible, during study design. Possible avenues for dealing with potential confounders include:

1. Match on potential confounders (see 'matching')

2. Collect data in a useful manner

3. Perform post-hoc analysis of these confounders.

In studies with small sample sizes, assessing confounding variables becomes very difficult because there is insufficient data to isolate data groupings and properly assess them.

Controls

Identifying the control group for a particular study is crucial for ensuring the usefulness and validity of study data. The ideal scenario is to use a true placebo but some useful studies compare the efficacy of competitive products aimed at achieving the same consumer result.

The traditional choice is to use an inactive placebo to measure the *background effect*. This background effect is used to measure the net effect of the product. For example, in a weight-loss product study, if those using the active product lost 7 pounds on average and the inactive placebo group lost 3 pounds, one would conclude that the real weight loss attributable to the product was 7 minus 3, or 4 pounds. The background effect is 3 pounds.

In other studies the placebo group may actually move in the opposite direction from the product group, thereby enhancing the product effect. In a joint mobility product study, the product subjects may report an improvement of 20 degrees while the placebo group may report a 3 degree reduction in their range-of-motion. The resulting 23 degree difference may help the product group achieve a statistically significant result.

Dosing Instructions

Dosing instructions used in the trial should be simple and are supposed to be the same as those printed on the labels and boxes of the actual product sold in the marketplace. A seasoned investigator can provide advice about how to word these instructions during the development phase. Any differences between the label and study instructions may cause the results to come into question.

Dropouts

Dropouts are subjects who begin the active phase of the trial and do not complete all the requirements (visits or outcome measures). The most common and frustrating reasons for subject dropout are lack of compliance with the study or not coming to follow-up visits. Other, less common reasons include serious adverse events such as accidents, medical conditions or illness. In the case of lack of compliance investigators may be tempted to try to persuade subjects to continue, however the Informed Consent requirements specify that human subject participation is voluntary—a subject is allowed to withdraw for no stated reason and may not be forced to continue against their will. The time, money and energy required to screen each subject is considerable, and the research incentive is to have as many of the enrolled subjects as possible finish the trial. Sometimes a financial incentive is provided but it is carefully monitored and subject to some debate by the IRB involved in each particular study.

An excessively high dropout rate may be considered a bias and subject the study to additional scientific scrutiny. As some studies are much more difficult than others, this is a vexing issue for both researchers and critics. A seasoned investigator must learn how to minimize this issue in his or her research.

Duration of Clinical Trial

The duration of the study is the duration (in days, weeks or months) of the active phase of the trial. In weight-loss studies the duration should be at least six weeks although some experts prefer trials lasting ten to twelve weeks. Research tells us that most people can make and sustain dietary or lifestyle changes for two to three weeks after which they tend to return to their normal habits. In order to reliably gauge whether a product related to these changes has a true effect, the active phase of a study must run longer than three weeks to compensate for this phenomenon.

Endpoints or Outcomes

The interchangeable terms *outcomes* or *endpoints* are what is being measured. Examples include weight, lipid values, erectile function, sleep quality and so forth.

It is generally agreed by experts that there should be only one main endpoint of the study with some secondary endpoints and safety endpoints included. Herbal or dietary supplement blends may affect a number of physiological systems and may seem appropriate for multiple outcomes. However, clinical trials maintain the highest validity and reliability when determining one primary outcome.

Using the optimal endpoint is a delicate balance that may involve medical equipment, laboratory testing, validated instrumentation and financial commitment.

When designing a study, the question of which outcome is the most appropriate and how it should be measured is a crucial determination leading to trial success.

Exclusion and Inclusion Criteria

These criteria define who will and will not be enrolled in the study. It is essential to think through the medical aspects of every trial in advance to avoid undermining the chances of success. The purpose of the trial is to support scientific claims, and these criteria will define the data available at the end of the trial.

As an example, in a study involving an adult weight-loss product, who are most likely to lose weight—women? Men? At what age? How does one deal with the fact that younger women may have an easier time losing weight but product marketing may be directed to middle-age women? An experienced investigator will know how to focus the study to maximize the usefulness of data available at the end of the trail.

Exclusion criteria: Subjects who give their informed consent are screened for the presence of criteria used to exclude them from the study. Exclusion criteria are designed to remove potential subjects from consideration for safety reasons or to eliminate the potential for other factors that may affect study outcomes. Candidates who meet the exclusion criteria do not go further in the study. The investigator screens each study candidate to ensure that the exclusion criteria are consistently and accurately applied. The development of exclusionary criteria is based on general safety concerns identified for particular medical conditions and the product being studied. A medical doctor may be retained to detect or confirm medical conditions. Samples might include subjects who:

- Are unwilling or unable to comply with any aspect of the clinical trial protocol;

- Are allergic to or express problems with ingredients in the active product or placebo;

- Have severe co-morbid condiitons (defined as any condition that would cause severe limitations or inability to carry out usual activities of daily living) including cardiac, pulmonary, renal or hepatic disease or active cancer;

- Use prescription or non-prescription products that may affect the process being studied;

- Consume alcohol at an elevated level;

- Are insulin dependent diabetics or have uncontrolled diabetes (as defined by A1c > 8);

- Have had surgery or a hospitalization within the past 3 months;

- Have a cardiovascular event;

- Have an acute illness;

- Have a Body Mass Index (BMI) of less than 25 or greater than 37.5 kg/m2;

- Have participated in a clinical trial in the past 4 weeks;

- Have any disease or condition that in the investigator's opinion compromises the integrity of the clinical trial or the safety of the subject;

- Women who are nursing, pregnant, or actively trying to become pregnant.

Inclusion criteria: Subjects who provide their informed consent are required to meet certain inclusion criteria specifically designed for the study. The investigator screens each study candidate to ensure the inclusionary criteria are consistently and accurately applied. Samples might include:

- Women and men who are overweight or obese (BMI > 25 and < 37.5 kg/m2) who wish to assess a beverage with the potential of assisting with appetite suppression and weight loss;
- Women and men who wish to promote healthy blood glucose management; or
- Women and men who are 18 to 70 years of age at the initial visit.

Formulations

There are many ingredients on the market today. Determining the precise blend or formula that is to be tested is an art based on the science of what properties each ingredient has been shown to provide and how they may interact with each other. When testing blended supplements, the exact formulation used in the clinical trial must be the same that is sold in the marketplace.

Free-Living

In a weight-loss study *free-living* refers to the instructions that subjects receive for a trial in which they are not placed on a specific diet or exercise program. They are asked to follow their normal diet and exercise patterns.

Hawthorne Effect

The term *Hawthorne Effect* was coined after a study involving industrial processing at the Hawthorne, Illinois, plant of AT&T's Western Electric Company. The Hawthorne Effect is when individuals in a study act differently simply because they are being observed. It can have such a powerful effect that techniques must be employed to ensure that it does not bias the study.

An example of the Hawthorne Effect can be seen in a diet study that requested subjects NOT to change their pre-study diet or exercise regimens. Individuals assigned to the placebo group may lose weight during the study simply due to conscious or subconscious seeds planted during a pre-study interview. As a result study participants make slight changes in the type of food they eat, the quantities they ingest and their level of physical activity. After detailed post-trial questioning following such a study with unexplained results, subjects will admit to making slight changes that affected the study outcome. A seasoned investigator is aware of this phenomenon and will take steps to minimize effects that can damage data usefulness.

Institutional Review Board (IRB) Approval

The primary role of an IRB is to protect subjects from unethical research. These boards work under Food and Drug Administration (FDA) guidelines and have circumscribed but strong powers.

An IRB works to protect the subject by assessing the research design using federal guidelines that cover such topics as the criteria for participation (both inclusionary and exclusionary criteria), laboratory testing and other aspects of the research protocol. Additionally, they review the informed consent that potential subjects will sign in order to participate. Like all organizations, IRBs have preferences and areas of interest. There are certain sections that they require and terminology they favor. Finally, their approval of all advertising and promotion (newspapers, radio, flyers, television or Internet-based) is required.

The role of the institutional review board has grown in recent decades but their origins go back to the human experimentation conducted by the Nazis during WWII and a few research projects in this country including the infamous Syphilis Trials. A summary of the issues involved in the American Syphilis Trials can be found in a *Science Magazine* article: "Uses and Abuses of Tuskegee" by Amy L. Fairchild and Ronald Bayer available on the website: www.sciencemag.org. (Fairchild and Bayer) Though we take subject safety for granted today, this was not the case years ago. The requirement that research be sponsored or approved by IRBs has greatly increased the safety and efficacy of dietary supplements and the benefits they claim to promote.

Seasoned investigator trials adhere to these requirements including, but not limited to, those listed below:

- The following FDA regulations should be incorporated into the conduct of research to assure that ethical standards will meet the worldwide rights of those subjects who participate in any study:
  - FDA Regulations 21 CRF Parts 50.20, 50.23, 50.25, 50.27, 54.1-54.6, 56.107-56.115, 312.50, 312.52, 312.53, 312.55-312.62, 312.66, 312.68-312.70.

- Studies should be conducted in compliance with Institutional Review Board/ Independent Ethics Committee (IRB/IEC) informed consent regulations and ICH GCP Guidelines.

- Studies should be conducted in compliance with all local regulatory requirements, in particular those which afford greater protection to the safety of the trial participants.

- All studies should be conducted according to the current revision of the Declaration of Helsinki (Revised South Africa 1996) and with local laws and regulations relevant to the use of new therapeutic agents in the country of conduct.

- Before initiating a trial an investigator/institution should have a written and dated approval/favorable opinion from the IRB for the trial protocol and/or amendment(s), a written informed consent form, consent form updates, subject recruitment procedures (e.g., advertisements) and written information to be provided to subjects.

Informed Consent

An investigator must obtain informed consent from each subject enrolled in the study in accordance with the U.S. Food and Drug Administration (FDA) regulation 21 CFR Parts 50.20-50.27 and the laws and regulations of the country in which the investigation is being conducted.

The IRB must approve the informed consent form and process to be used by the investigator. This includes ensuring that the subject has the legal and mental capacity to form intent and that they confirm their intent by signing a form. The investigator is responsible for ensuring that informed consent is obtained from the subject before any research activity is undertaken. This includes any diagnostic or therapeutic procedures as well as the administration of the initial dose of the study medication.

Matching Variables

One mechanism design experts use in minimizing potential study bias is to match study groups on certain variables. Specific variables will be controlled to be similar in both the treatment and control experimental groups. For example, by matching on sex (e.g., only women will be eligible), the groups are more similar. In a diet study, we might choose to have only female subjects in the study. The upside of including only females is that the population is more consistent, but the downside is that we cannot assess men with this study. Although this seems obvious in the case of gender, there are many other variables to consider which may not be as obvious or clear. Other matching variables might include age (within 5 years), BMI (Body Mass Index), or the presence of certain medical conditions.

Pharmaceutical-Level Clinical Trials

Describing a trial as *pharmaceutical-level* means that it meets the higher-order Gold-Standard criteria applied to the pharmaceutical industry. There are significant differences between non-pharmaceutical and pharmaceutical-level trials, including some or all of the following parameters:

- Appropriate design expertise

- Appropriate controls

- IRB-approval

- Sample sizes

- Attention to potential biases (selection, Hawthorne Effect, misclassification and others)

- Endpoints

- Laboratory work

- Independent scientific oversight

- Subject reimbursement

- Duration of the study

- Lack of a run-in period

- Lack of various medical professionals (physicians, nurses, dietitians, respiratory therapists, etc.)

- Lack of independent biostatisticians for the analysis phase

- Lack of sophisticated medical measurement equipment

Placebo

A *placebo* is a product that looks identical to the actual product being tested but contains none of the active ingredients. The placebo must simulate the actual product in appearance while delivering a non-physiological effect. It must look, taste, and otherwise appear as if it could actually be the real product. It may NOT be a capsule with ingredients that couldn't pass the "straight-face test." If the real product is a blend of many different herbs and vitamin ingredients one would expect a multi-colored and multi-textured placebo. It must be made so that a subject couldn't discern if they took it apart if it was the product or the placebo. The manufacturing of reasonable placebo samples may require an experienced manufacturer and may add a level of complexity.

Placebo-Controlled

The term *placebo-controlled* refers to the type of study in which a placebo group is compared to a group receiving the actual product.

Novices often wonder why a placebo or control group is necessary given that it drives up the cost of the study and may seem to diminish the effect of the product. However, in certain studies failure to use a valid control group (that is on a placebo) will mean that the results of the study are less valid and will be questioned.

A study that does NOT use a control is called an *open-label study*, defined by the fact that the subjects and staff KNOW that they are taking product. This type of study is appropriate in some situations. (See the section "Types of Studies or Trials.")

In a weight-loss study the weight loss experienced by the placebo group should be subtracted from the product group. If the average weight loss in the placebo group was three (3) pounds and the weight loss in the product group was nine (9) pounds for the same period, then the actual weight loss due to the product would be six (6) pounds. Without the control or placebo group, one might inappropriately conclude that the product was responsible for an average weight loss of the full nine (9) pounds. When offering this product to consumers, an expectation of nine pounds of average weight loss is unrealistic and could lead to adverse consumer claims. Controls are employed to ensure we are measuring the true effect of the product. Without the control, the nine pounds is merely an estimate.

There are times when the placebo group performs worse, making the actual effect that much stronger. In a study of an anti-aging product using 70-year-old men, several endpoints in the placebo group were reported as less-improved or weaker over the course of 4 months. The product group reported improved numbers over baseline, strengthening the effect of the product and helping make the product results statistically significant.

Randomization

Randomization describes the way in which subjects are assigned to the treatment/product group or control (placebo or other type of control) group. In a randomized study, neither subjects nor staff conducting the study know which group subjects are in AND each subject has an equal chance of ending up in either group. Study experts use randomization as a time-tested method to ensure that the results are valid. Since neither subjects nor the staff know the group assignment, subject responses are more likely to be their true responses.

Precise randomization methodologies are employed using "blocks." In studies involving two groups (product and placebo), blocks of six (6) or eight (8) are typically used. From every six (6) subjects equal numbers will be assigned to both groups. In this manner the overall numbers of the two groups will always be similar. In studies involving three groups, such as two products and a placebo, a block size involves a multiple of three such as nine (9) or twelve (12). Standard randomization charts are used to determine the assignments, ensuring that all subjects have an equal chance of being assigned to the various groups.

Run-in Period

Run-in periods are short time frames at the beginning of a study used to establish baselines and test the compliance of new subjects. Run-in periods are typically one to two weeks in duration, but sometimes last longer when it is critical to develop laboratory baselines. They are useful for establishing more precise baselines and to weed out noncompliant subjects. The downside is that they increase the cost of a study.

Sample Size

The *sample size* refers to the number of subjects required to complete a study in order to reasonably expect to be able to document an existing difference. These numbers are derived from statistical calculations made during the design phase and involve a number of assumptions. They include such variables as the expected level of the primary outcome achieved by both the treatment and placebo groups and the chance of detecting a difference if one exists. Entire chapters of advanced statistical theory have been devoted to these issues. Readers who wish to explore these and other statistical topics should consult a technical resource or a reputable research firm.

Statistical Significance

Statistical significance is typically established at 0.05. This means that the differences one observes between the placebo and product results have a 5 percent chance of occurring randomly. It is thought that a one in twenty chance virtually assures that the results (if different) are "real" and not due to chance alone.

Study Design Types

The *study design* is a blueprint that defines the study structure. It provides all the basic principles and parameters and defines research strategies. An investigator must make informed choices in putting a study together. There are three major study structures:

Parallel-Group: In this study there are two or more groups where subjects are randomized to one of the groups and are followed for the duration of the study;

Crossover: In this design, subjects start in one group (product or placebo/control) and are followed for a specified time period. At a set point, there is a short washout period during which they don't take any product, and then switch over to the other group (if they start on product, they switch to placebo, or vice versa). In this case, each subject acts as his or her own control. The advantage of this approach is that fewer subjects are needed to achieve statistical significance. The disadvantage is that the study takes more than twice as long to complete. The costs are about the same, but some product categories are better for crossover designs.

Open-Label: In an open-label trial, both the subjects and staff know that they are taking product and no placebo or control is involved.

Subject Compensation

Compensation is an amount in dollars paid to subjects who complete the trial. Typically in dietary supplement trials subjects receive between $100 and $200 based on the trial difficulty and duration. Even at $100, if the trial involves 60 subjects to complete, this is a $6,000 budgetary item.

The amount and terms of the compensation are determined by the IRB involved in the trial. In cases involving partial completion, some IRBs require payment per visit regardless of the usefulness of the data obtained. This is particularly onerous because money is spent on data that may not end up contributing to study outcomes.

Types of Studies or Trials

Marketing Studies

The purpose of a *marketing study* generally includes soft endpoints which involve subjective criteria (taste, texture, appeal) rather than actual efficacy-type endpoints (blood levels, weight loss, etc.) that may involve some of the following parameters. Examples of soft endpoints are:

- Taste
- Texture
- Aroma
- Sensation
- Usefulness
- Delivery system
- Efficacy

Marketing studies may be conducted once clinical trial research has confirmed a particular endpoint to aid in positioning the product with consumers or to refine a marketing campaign that has fallen short of plans and goals. These studies are not required to meet industry standards for human-subject research.

Pilot Clinical Trials (Proof-of-Concept)

A *pilot trial* is the same as a full trial except that it differs in the sample size. A pilot trial may be completed with only a quarter or a third of the numbers required to demonstrate statistical significance in a full trial. Companies often begin the process by ordering a pilot trial in order to conserve funds and to increase the chance of generating useful data in a larger trial. Another common use of a pilot trial is to test two or three different blends to determine which is more efficacious, and thus should undergo further testing.

Companies sometimes use pilots as a way of financing full trials. If the results are solid, companies can use them to secure additional funding to complete the full trial.

Generally speaking, pilot trials are useful to demonstrate how products will react for specific endpoints but lack the sample size required to achieve statistical significance. Depending on how the pilot is designed, these data may or may not be used in the full trial.

These are some of the reasons companies might begin with a pilot trial, then proceed to a full trial, which offers regulatory protection.

Product Testing

Product testing refers to a laboratory test of the blend or product. Companies are often interested in certifying the precise details of their blend in order to validate the blending procedure. Questions regarding the quality of the manufacturing process can be answered to some degree through a paper trail but full verification requires the work of an experienced laboratory. Blends can be tested against the paper-trail documentation such as receipts, packing slips and labels. This information lends support to a company's marketing claims and facilitates sound decision making regarding which raw ingredients to use in the future.

Laboratories are located throughout the country and can be found through referrals from industry consultants. Companies may require the advice of an experienced and perhaps independent research scientist to interpret the data. This depends upon the laboratory and how its reports are developed.

Open-Label Trials

An *open-label trial* is where both the subjects and staff know that the subjects are taking the actual product. In these cases, there is no placebo or control involved.

Open-label trials are used either in the pilot phase or in the case in which the biology of the product makes a control less of an issue. In the case of a product being assessed for enzymatic activity, one can employ an open-label approach by taking baseline levels, giving the product designed to change enzyme levels, then measuring after the desired duration has been achieved. A disadvantage of open-label trials is that they are considered less of a gold standard. The primary advantage is budgetary.

The Gold-Standard Design: Randomized, Placebo-Controlled, Blinded Clinical Trial

A gold-standard clinical trial is a pharmaceutical-level type trial employing a control group, IRB approval, randomization, blinding, oversight, and more. The name comes from the idea that all strategies that can improve validity and reliability are employed together. Embedded in this category is the type of study that can include parallel or crossover design features.

Randomized, placebo-controlled, blinded trials are those that typically decide if a new drug will make it into the marketplace and are generally reported in scientific literature. For a new drug, the FDA has defined four levels of required trials involving efficacy and safety and multi-site studies. Each may require months or years of planning, execution and analysis. In addition, at any point throughout the process the drug may require changes in the following areas:

- Dosing or delivery;
- The identification or definition of contraindication;
- Changes in the endpoints;
- Changes in the laboratory values; and
- Other parameters.

This is an important contributing factor as to why only a fraction of all drugs make it through the FDA process and become licensed.

There is obviously higher cost associated with the increase in scientific credibility. Costs can be in the millions of dollars.

All gold-standard trials include:

- Randomization
- Placebo-Control
- Blinding
- Physician oversight
- Bi-weekly status reports

  Discretionary options are:

- Independent statistical analysis
- Independent study oversight
- Laboratory testing
- Special medical testing
- Resting metabolic rate
- Body fat and lean muscle mass (as measured using Life Measurement, Inc.'s Bod Pod)
- Computerized neurocognitive testing

Post-Trial Activities

Statistical Analysis

Careful and systematic analysis of study findings is essential to understand the nature of consumer benefit, to develop supportable claims and to identify future problems. An individual with proper credentials and training in supplement research is required to conduct the review of research findings and isolate the important findings upon which one may rely.

Publishing Trial Results

Most important research results are published in some form to support the advancement of medical industry knowledge. This is research that other scientists rely on and that supplement companies use to determine which ingredients and blends to market. Publishing helps to promote public safety because results are available to other scientists and the general public. Knowing about poor results or adverse events from other studies can save money and prevent suffering. Finally, publishing results in reputable journals lends credibility to the results.

Research Funding

In some cases, state and federal funding is available to conduct follow-up research to confirm questionable findings or to study a new area identified through a completed study. Securing grant opportunities is a long-range strategy because this process may take several years to get off the ground, but the rewards are increased credibility and subsequent marketing opportunities.

Legal Action

Federal Trade Commission (FTC) law requires advertising claims to be supported by science. It is not sufficient to rely on existing data. If a product makes claims associated with sexual health, weight loss or sleep quality, all considered health matters, then both the individual ingredients and the 'blend' require substantiation.

Existing medical conditions of study subjects can also be the cause for costly legal action. Experienced researchers know how to identify and control for these concerns. Review of past research prior to clinical testing as well as vigilance about the most common contra-indicated medical conditions during the trial prevents costly legal claims. Ethical considerations may require removing ingredients while in the production stage and/or the use of proper label warnings to protect consumers.

Lawsuits, regulatory fines and lost consumer confidence are costly and can have long lasting negative effects on a company's ability to continue sales or develop new products to keep up with new developments. Many companies learn this lesson the hard way.

Sources

"Bias." *Wikipedia*. http://www.wikipedia.com (accessed July, 2007).

Elston, R. C., and Johnson, W. D. *Essentials of Biostatistics*, 2nd edition. Philadelphia: F.A. Davis Company, 1994.

"Epidemiology" *Wikipedia*. http://www.wikipedia.com, (accessed July, 2007).

Fairchild, A. L., and R. Bayer. *Uses and Abuses of Tuskegee*. May 1999, Vol. 284. no. 5416, pp 919-921, by *Science Magazine*. Accessed on sciencemag.com July 2007.

Friis, R. H., and T. A. Sellers. *Epidemiology for Public Health Practice*. Boston: Jones and Bartlett Publishers, 2004.

Gordis, L. *Epidemiology*, 2nd edition. Philadelphia: W.B. Saunders Company, 2000.

Greenberg, Raymond S. et al. *Medical Epidemiology*. New York: Lange Medical Books/McGraw-Hill, 2001.

Hulley, Stephen, B. and Cummings, Steven R. *Designing Clinical Research*. Baltimore: Williams and Wilkens, 1988.

Lilienfeld, Abraham M. and David, *Foundations of Epidemiology*, 3rd edition. New York: Oxford University Press, 1988.

Meinert, Curtis L. Clinical Trials: Design, Conduct, and Analysis. New York: Oxford University Press, 1986.

"Scientific Method" Merriam Webster's Online Dictionary. http://www.m-w.com/dictionary/scientific%20method (accessed July, 2007).

"Scientific Method" *Wikipedia*. http://www.wikipedia.com (accessed July, 2007).

Sokal, Robert R. and Rohlf, F. James. *Biometry*, 2nd edition. New York: W.H. Freeman and Company, 1980.

About the Author

James M. Blum is an epidemiologist and principal consultant of DSRG with 37 years of experience in both the medical field and dietary supplement research.

Index

To order additional copies of
Feed Your Brain Lose Your Belly
or the weight loss product Vi-texxa™,
please go to www.Vi-texxa.com.